MOLECULAR BIOLOGY AND GENETICS OF CHILDHOOD CANCERS:
Approaches to Neuroblastoma

Ellis Horwood books in the
BIOLOGICAL SCIENCES
General Editor: Dr ALAN WISEMAN, University of Surrey, Guildford

Series in
BIOCHEMISTRY AND BIOTECHNOLOGY
Series Editor: Dr ALAN WISEMAN, Senior Lecturer in the Division of Biochemistry, University of Surrey, Guildford

Aitken, J.	**Handbook of Enzyme Active Site Identification***
Ambrose, E.J.	**The Nature and Origin of the Biological World**
Austin, B. & Brown, C.M.	**Microbial Biotechnology: Freshwater and Marine Environments***
Berkeley, R.C.W., *et al.*	**Microbial Adhesion to Surfaces**
Bertoncello, I.	**Human Cell Cultures for Screening Anti-Cancer Rays***
Blackburn, F. & Knapp, J.S.	**Agricultural Microbiology***
Bowen, W.R.	**Membrane Separation Processes***
Bubel, A. & Fitzsimons, C.	**Microstructure and Function of Cells**
Clarke, C.R. & Moos, W. H.	**Drug Discovery Technologies***
Cooke, N.	**Potassium Channels***
Corkill, J.A.	**Clinical Biochemistry: The Analysis of Biologically-Important Compounds and Drugs***
Crabbe, M.J.C.	**Enzyme Biotechnology and Protein Engineering**
Crabbe, M.J.C.	**Kinetics of Enzymes***
Denyer, S. & Baird, R.	**Handbook of Microbiological Control***
Dolly, J.O.	**Neurotoxins in Neurochemistry**
Espinal, J.	**Understanding Insulin Action***
Eyzaguirre, J.	**Chemical Modification of Enzymes**
Eyzaguirre, J.	**Human Biochemistry and Molecular Biology***
Ferencik, M.	**Immunochemistry***
Fish, N.M.	**Computer Applications in Fermentation Technology***
Francis, J.L.	**Haemostasis and Cancer***
Gemeiner, P. *et al.*	**Enzyme Engineering***
Harding, J.	**Biochemistry and Pharmacology of Cataract Research: Drug Therapy Approaches***
Horobin, R.W.	**Understanding Histochemistry: Selection, Evaluation and Design of Biological Stains**
Hudson, M.J. & Pyle, P.L.	**Separations for Biotechnology, Vol 2***
Hughes, J.	**The Neuropeptide CCK***
Inoki, R., Kudo T. & Olgart, L.M.	**Dynamic Aspects of Dental Pulp***
Jordan, T.W.	**Fungal Toxins and Chemistry***
Junter, G.A.	**Electrochemical Detection Techniques in the Applied Biosciences: Vol. 1: Analysis and Clinical Applications Vol. 2: Fermentation and Bioprocess Control, Hygiene and Environmental Sciences**
Kennedy, J.F. & White, C.A.	**Bioactive Carbohydrates**
Krcmery, V.	**Antibiotic and Chemotherapeutic Compounds***
Palmer, T.	**Understanding Enzymes, 2nd Edition**
Paterson, R.	**Biological Applications of Membranes**
Reizer, J. & Peterkofsky, A.	**Sugar Transport and Metabolism in Gram-positive Bacteria**
Russell, N. J.	**Microbes and Temperature***
Russell, N.J. & Gacesa, P.	**Pseudomonas Infection and Alginates: Structures, Properties and Functions in Pathogenesis***
Scragg, A.H.	**Biotechnology for Engineers: Biological Systems in Technological Processes**
Sikyta, B.	**Methods in Industrial Microbiology**
Sluyser, M.	**Molecular Biology of Cancer Genes**
Sluyser, M. & Voûte, P.A.	**Molecular Biology and Genetics of Childhood Cancers: Approaches to Neuroblastoma**
Verrall, M.S.	**Discovery and Isolation of Microbial Prodoucts**
Verrall, M.S. & Hudson, M.J.	**Separations for Biotechnology**
Webb, C. & Mavituna, F.	**Plant and Animal Cells: Process Possibilities**
Winkler, M.	**Biochemical Process Engineering***
Wiseman, A.	**Handbook of Enzyme Biotechnology, 2nd Edition**
Wiseman, A.	**Topics in Enzyme and Fermentation Biotechnology Vols. 1, 2, 4, 6, 8**
Wiseman, A.	**Enzyme Induction, Mutagen Activation and Carcinogen Testing in Yeast**
Wiseman, A.	**Genetically Engineered Proteins and Enzymes from Yeasts***

* *In preparation*

MOLECULAR BIOLOGY AND GENETICS OF CHILDHOOD CANCERS:
Approaches to Neuroblastoma

Editors:
M. SLUYSER
Division of Tumour Biology
Netherlands Cancer Institute
and
A. VOÛTE
Specialist in Child Oncology
Emma Kinderzeikenhuis, Amsterdam

ELLIS HORWOOD LIMITED
Publishers · Chichester

Halsted Press: a division of
JOHN WILEY & SONS
New York · Chichester · Brisbane · Toronto

First published in 1988 by
ELLIS HORWOOD LIMITED
Market Cross House, Cooper Street,
Chichester, West Sussex, PO19 1EB, England
The publisher's colophon is reproduced from James Gillison's drawing of the ancient Market Cross, Chichester.

Distributors:
Australia and New Zealand:
JACARANDA WILEY LIMITED
GPO Box 859, Brisbane, Queensland 4001, Australia
Canada:
JOHN WILEY & SONS CANADA LIMITED
22 Worcester Road, Rexdale, Ontario, Canada
Europe and Africa:
JOHN WILEY & SONS LIMITED
Baffins Lane, Chichester, West Sussex, England
North and South America and the rest of the world:
Halsted Press: a division of
JOHN WILEY & SONS
605 Third Avenue, New York, NY 10158, USA
South-East Asia
JOHN WILEY & SONS (SEA) PTE LIMITED
37 Jalan Pemimpin # 05–04
Block B, Union Industrial Building, Singapore 2057
Indian Subcontinent
WILEY EASTERN LIMITED
4835/24 Ansari Road
Daryaganj, New Delhi 110002, India

British Library Cataloguing in Publication Data
Molecular Biology and Genetics of Childhood Cancers: Approaches to Neuroblastoma
1. Children. Nervous system. Neuroblastomas. Diagnosis. Applications of molecular genetics
I. Sluyser, M. (Mels) *1930–* II. Voûte, A.
618.92′9948075

Library of Congress Card No. 88–24358

ISBN 0–7458–0547–7 (Ellis Horwood Limited)
ISBN 0–470–21237–3 (Halsted Press)

Typeset in Times by Ellis Horwood Limited
Printed in Great Britain by Hartnolls, Bodmin

Table of contents

1

General introduction

P. A. Voûte
Department of Nuclear Medicine and Werkgroep Kindertumoren, The Netherlands Cancer Institute, 1066 CX Amsterdam, The Netherlands

1 INTRODUCTION

A neuroblastoma is a tumour from the sympathetic nervous system. Other tumours occurring in the sympathetic nervous system are ganglioneuroma and phaeochromocytoma. All three arise from the same embryonic tissue and have the same anatomical sites. The tumour is derived from the ventrally migrating cells of the neurocrest. The ventrally migrating cells develop normally into the spinal ganglia, the ganglia of the sympathetic side-chain, the prevertebral ganglia, the paraganglia and the chromaffin bodies as well as APUD cells and the leptomeninges. The cells migrating from the neural crest, which form the sympathetic nervous system, are called sympathetic neuroblasts or sympathogonia. The sympathogonia migrate further to the adrenal medulla and the retroperitoneal ganglia along the aorta. These sympathogonia are pluripotential cells and they can differentiate into chromaffin cells, neurofibrous cells and sympathetic ganglion cells [1].

The anatomical sites of the sympathetic nervous system indicate where tumours of this system can be found (Figs 1 and 2). They occur in the sympathetic side-chain from the base of the skull to deep in the pelvis, in the adrenals and in the retroperitoneal paraganglia. These retroperitoneal paraganglia are in newborns the most important source for noradrenalin production. Neuroblastomas are found for 5% of the cases in the pelvic sympathetic side-chain, 17% in the thorax and 8% in the cervical sympathetic side-chain. 70% of the cases originate in the retroperitoneal region; in 30% the probable site of origin is the adrenal gland and in 10% the abdominal sympathetic side-chain.

2. PATHOLOGY

In neuroblastoma intermediate stages in the development of sympathogonia to ganglion cells to neurofibrous cells and chromaffin cells can be found. Depending on

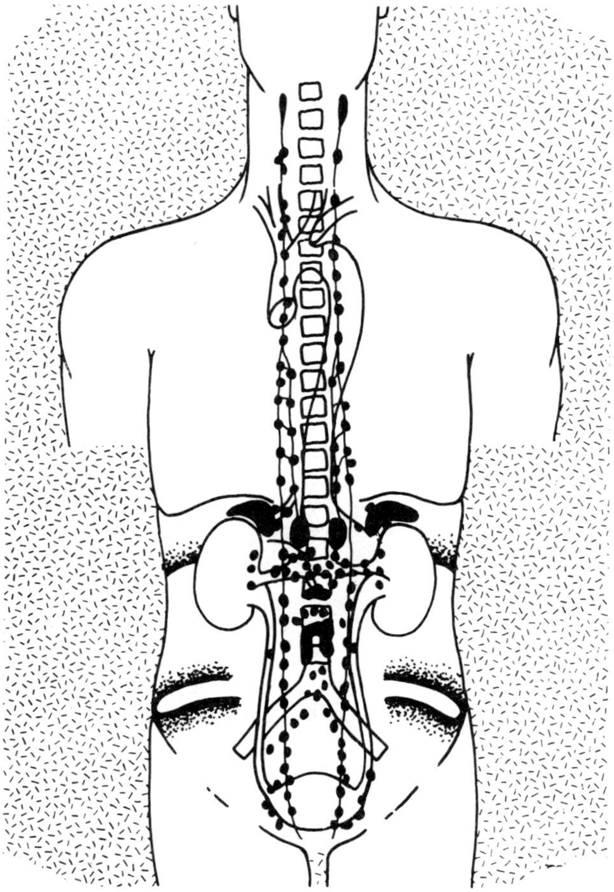

Fig. 1 — Schematic anatomical localization of the sympathetic nervous system.

the number of intermediate stages, the tumours have received names such as sympathicoblastoma, ganglioneuroma or ganglioneuroblastoma. Neuroblastoma was originally described as a glia-cell tumour. The fast-growing neuroblastoma is made up of closely packed sympathogonia, without any differentiation; the cell type corresponds to the migrating sympathogonia in the sympathetic trunk. The first indication of organization is a grouping of the cells in rosette-like arrangements. Delicate nerve fibres can emerge from the precursors of the ganglion cells, and these fibres intertwine to form the centre of each rosette. A neuroblastoma is a tumour made up of sympathogonia which multiply much as they do during the embryonic period. Some differentiate into rosettes and ganglion cells and others into immature chromaffin cells. By virtue of its origin, a neuroblastoma has the potential ability to mature into either ganglioneuromas or phaeochromocytomas. Attempts have been made to correlate the histological grade of neuroblastomas with their biological behaviour. Vesicular nuclei, cytoplasm and cytoplasmic processes, the presence of mature ganglion cells, and probably rosette formation suggest increasing maturity

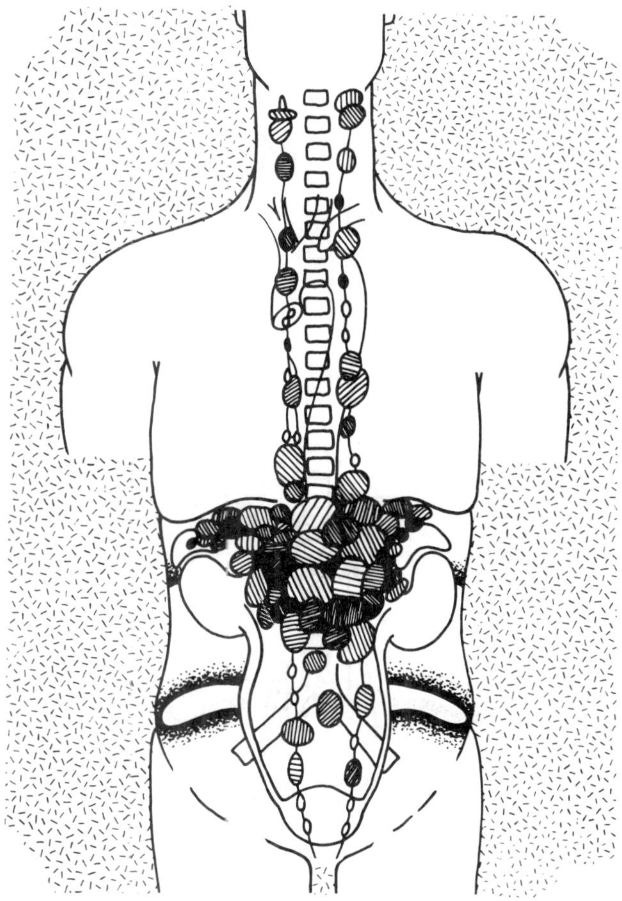

Fig. 2 — Localization of neuroblastomas imposed on the sympathetic nervous system.

and are associated with a favourable prognosis. There is a spectrum ranging from a tumour composed of cells so completely undifferentiated that their distinction from the other small round tumours of childhood is almost impossible to a tumour composed of mature ganglion cells.

Neuroblastomas can occur congenitally, even with placental metastases. Of all patients 50% are younger than 2 years and 75% younger than 4 years. The tumour is exceedingly rare after the age of 14. Neuroblastomas can occur familially, but this is rare. Occasionally neuroblastomas are mentioned in families with phaeochromocytomas and ganglioneuromas.

3. CLINICAL MANIFESTATIONS

There is a wide range of symptoms of neuroblastoma, which is partly due to the numerous sites of the primary tumour. It is also due to the wide pattern of metastases and to the symptoms that can be attributed to the associated metabolic and immunological disturbances in the body. In the neck and head region a palpable mass and Horner's syndrome (Fig. 3) can be the first symptoms. In the chest the tumour

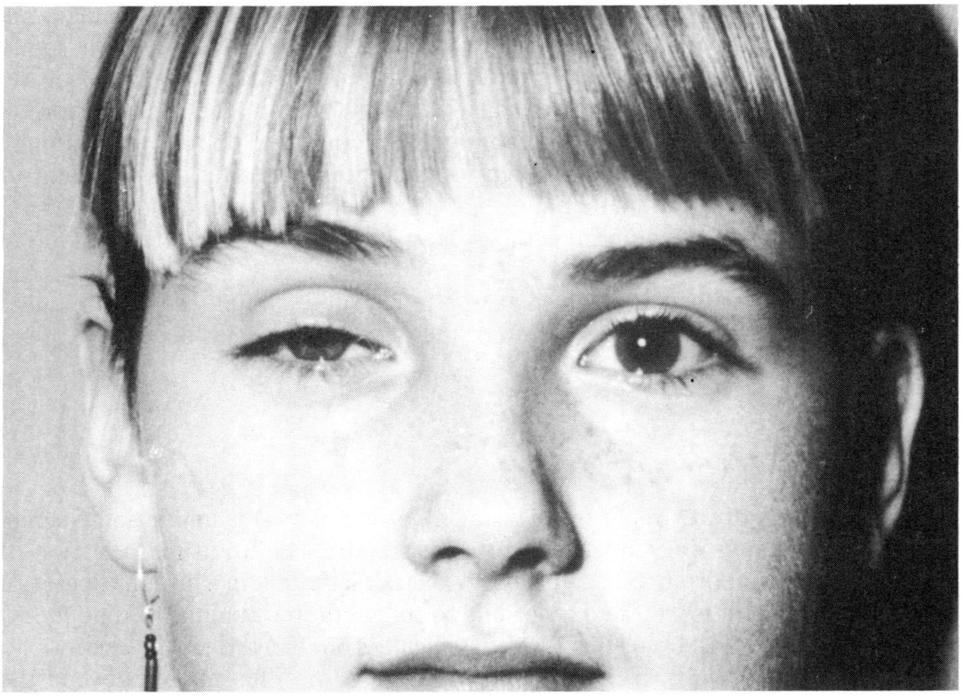

Fig. 3 — Horner's syndrome, miosis, ptosis and endophthalmitis associated with a neuroblastoma in the cervical sympathetic side-chain.

can give rise to respiratory distress, dysphagia and circulatory problems. Abdominal pain and a palpable mass will be the signs for an abdominal tumour. Pelvic tumours will give rise to problems of defaecation and voiding. When a tumour develops in the sympathetic side-chain the neuroblastoma can be of the dumb-bell or the hour-glass type. The signs of compression of the spinal cord depend on the location of the tumour.

Metabolic signs can occur as a result of the excessive production and excretion of catecholamines. These signs are hypertension, flushing and periods of excessive sweating. In some neuroblastomas watery diarrhoea with atonic bowel and extreme loss of potassium can occur, as an effect of the so-called vaso-active intestinal peptide (VIP), a neurotransmitter hormone. Immunological symptoms can occur in the form of neurological problems due to encephalopathy, characterized by ataxia and opsomyoclonus. This phenomenon is thought to be some kind of an auto-immune response, with an evoked immune reaction to the tumour which then is directed to the normal brain tissue.

The clinical symptoms of metastases will vary widely. In young babies the diffuse liver metastases can lead to an enlarged liver and can give rise to a prolonged jaundice and circulatory problems. Subcutaneous metastases, nodules with a bluish colour, may be the presenting sign. The older age group shows a different pattern of metastatic spread. The difference is due to the change in circulation from the foetal circulation to the circulation of the newborn. In the older age group, skeletal, bone marrow and lymph node metastases are predominant. Some organs, i.e. brain, spinal cord, heart and lungs, are virtually never the site of metastases. Invasion of the paratesticular spermatic cord is seen fairly often, but chromaffin tissue is normal tissue around the spermatic cord. Laboratory findings are due to the enlarged excretion of dopametabolites. Although some authors state that it is sufficient to determine only one or two metabolites, this is not the correct procedure [2]. It is of the utmost importance to determine the wide variety of different metabolites of the dopametabolism.

Some patients with neuroblastoma excrete elevated amounts of cystathionine and homocystine in the urine [3]. Both of these two amino acids occur in nervous tissue as well as in the liver.

4. CLINICAL STAGING

In the evaluation of treatment results, staging of the disease is important. Staging provides information relevant to the prognosis and is helpful in the selection of treatment. Most important for staging is the TNM description, in which the degree of tumour involvement is stratified according to three criteria: tumour (T), node (N) and metastases (M) [4]. Using this TNM classification one can arrive at a description.

Primary tumour (T): since it is often impossible to differentiate between the primary tumour and the adjacent lymph nodes, the T assessment relates to the total mass. When there is doubt about multiple primaries or metastases, the latter are presumed. The tumour classification is as follows:

T0 no evidence of primary tumour
T1 single tumour, 5 cm or less in its greatest dimension
T2 single tumour, more than 5 cm but not more than 10 cm in its greatest dimension
T3 single tumour, more than 10 cm in its greatest dimension
T4 multiple tumours occurring simultaneously
Tx the minimum requirements to assess the primary tumour cannot be met

Regional lymph nodes (N) are classified as follows:

N0 no evidence of regional lymph node involvement
N1 evidence of regional lymph node involvement
Nx the minimum requirements to assess the regional lymph nodes cannot be met

Distant metastases (M) are classified as follows:

M0 no evidence of distant metastases

M1 evidence of distant metastases
Mx the minimum requirements to assess distant metastases cannot be met

The criteria are grouped into stages:

Stage	TNM classification		
Stage I	T1	N0Nx	M0
Stage II	T2	N0Nx	M0
Stage III	T1T2	any N1	M0
	T3	any N	M0
Stage IV	T1T2T3	any N	M1
Stage V	T4	any N	any M

This TNM staging is based on physical and clinical investigations at diagnosis. CT scanning and NMR imaging are making this highly reliable. There is also a p-TNM staging based on surgical and pathological findings.

5. CONCLUSIONS

New approaches to diagnosis seem also to lead to new thoughts about treatment. The monoclonal antibodies can play an important part in distinguishing neuroblastoma from other small round cell tumours of childhood. The rapidly developing specialities of molecular biology and cytogenetics will certainly have an impact on the diagnosis, the treatment and the prognosis.

There is a need for better diagnostic tests and for new approaches to treatment. More has to be learned about the control of growth and it is hoped that biological response modifiers will begin to play a role in the treatment of neuroblastoma in the future [5].

REFERENCES

[1] Coupland, R. E. (1965). *The Natural history of the Chromaffin Cell,* Longman, London

[2] Abeling, N. G., van Gennip, A. H., Overmars, H. & Voûte, P. A. (1986). Biochemical monitoring of children with neuroblastoma. *Radiother. Oncol.* **7** 27–35

[3] Rajnherc, J. R., van Gennip, A. H., Abeling, N. G. G. M., van der Zee, J. M. & Voûte, P. A. (1984). Cystathioninuria in patients with neuroblastoma. *Med. Pediatr. Oncol.* **12** 81–84

[4] UICC (1985). *TNM-atlas, Illustrated Guide to the TNM/pTNM-Classification of Malignant Tumours,* 2nd end., UICC, Geneva

[5] Voûte, P. A., de Kraker, J. & Burgers, J. M. V. (1986). Tumours of the sympathetic nervous system. In: P. A. Voûte, A. Barrett *et al.* (eds.) *Cancer in Children,* 2nd edn., Springer Verlag, Heidelberg, New York

2

Tumour markers in neuroblastoma

Jacques Ninane, Christiane Vermylen and **Guy Cornu**
Department of Paediatric Haematology and Oncology, Cliniques Universitaires Saint-Luc, 10 avenue Hippocrate, B-1200 Brussels, Belgium

A marker is a dream for a paediatric oncologist. The ideal tumour marker would be a specific molecule produced by the malignant cell, measurable at the time of diagnosis, absent during periods of remission, and present once more in relapse. Unfortunately, in neuroblastoma, few markers meet these stringent criteria. Some cellular markers, such as antigens detected by monoclonal antibodies, oncogenes and radiolabelled MIBG — a structural analogue of guanethidine with certain structural similarities to norepinephrine — are treated in other sections of this book. In this chapter four 'circulating' markers of neuroblastoma, detectable either in patients' blood or in their urine, will be discussed: catecholamines, neuron-specific enolase, ferritin and gangliosides.

1. CATECHOLAMINES

In 1959, excessive secretion of vanillylmandelic acid (VMA) was noticed in children with ganglioneuroma [1] and ganglioneuroblastoma [2]. In the next two years, increased urinary excretion of dopamine (DA) and 3,4-dihydroxyphenylalanine (DOPA) were reported as being associated with neuroblastoma [3]. Today the fact that neuroblastoma cells secrete large amounts of one or more catecholamines, as well as their metabolites, is well documented.

Despite the fact that VMA and homovanillic acid (HVA) are two metabolites that are relatively easy to measure and the most frequently elevated in neuroblastoma, there are 'non-secreting' tumours for which less frequently measured metabolites may be useful in establishing the diagnosis. It is therefore important to have a good understanding of the synthesis and metabolism of catecholamines, their precursors and their intermediate products although, for practical clinical purposes, HVA and VMA are the most widely used in the diagnosis and follow-up of children with neuroblastoma (Fig. 1).

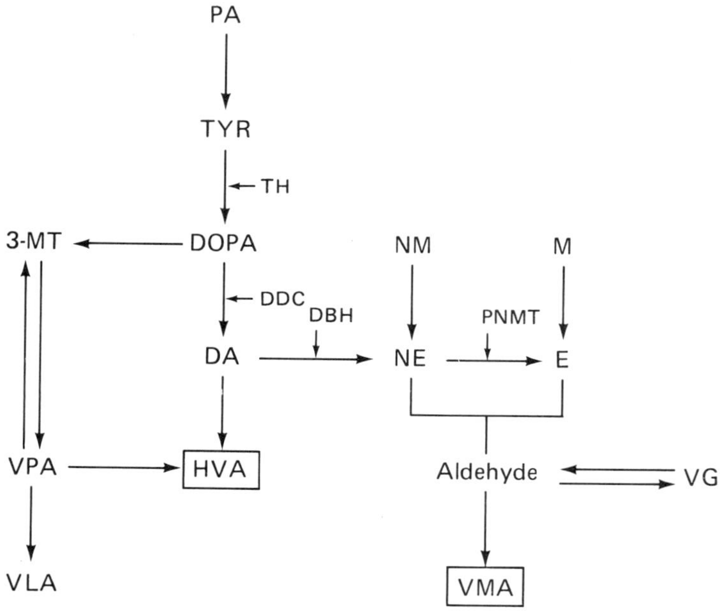

Fig. 1 — Metabolism of catecholamines. *Enzymes:* TH (tyrosine hydroxylase), DDC (dopa-decarboxylase), PNMT (phenylethanolamine-*N*-methyl transferase), DBH (dopamine-β-hydroxylase). *Catecholamines, metabolites and precursors:* PA (phenylalanine), TYR (tyrosine), DOPA (3,4-dihydroxylphenylalanine), DA (dopamine), NE (norepinephrine), E (epinephrine), VMA (vanillylmandelic acid), HVA (homovanillic acid), NM (normetanephrine), M (methanephrine), MT (3-methoxytyramine), VLA (vanillactic acid), VPA (vanilpuric acid), VG (vanilglycol).

1.1 Urinary HVA and VMA levels

During the past 20 years the measurement of urinary VMA and HVA has become a routine test for diagnosis and follow-up of patients with neuroblastoma.

Several methods have been used including, among others, bidirectional paper chromatography [4], high-voltage electrophoresis [3] and, more recently, high performance liquid chromatography [5] or capillary gas chromatography [6].

1.1.1 Random samples of 24 h collections?

The classical methodology stated that a 24 h urine collection was necessary and most authors still recommend it as the only way to obtain reliable and comparable data. This statement has recently been challenged by Tuchman and coworkers: they showed not only that random urinary HVA and VMA levels were adequate for utilization in the diagnosis of neuroblastoma but, moreover, that sequential determination of random HVA and VMA were helpful in the follow-up of those patients [7]. A three-year study performed by the same authors led them to conclude that prolonged urine collections for HVA and VMA determinations in the diagnosis of neuroblastoma are no longer necessary [8]. In view of their data, it seems quite possible to dispense with 24 h urine collections, which, especially in young children, are difficult to obtain and time consuming.

1.1.2 Mass screening for neuroblastoma

One of the most important problems in neuroblastoma is the treatment of advanced stages in children older than 12 months. Although, thanks to intensive chemotherapy, the number of long-term survivors has increased over the past decade [9], too many children with stage IV neuroblastoma eventually die from their disease when they are diagnosed over one year of age.

In contrast, about 80% of babies under one year are probably curable. It then seemed logical to try to detect neuroblastoma in its early stage, especially during infancy. Since 1973, Sawada and his colleagues have organized in Kyoto, Japan, what they call a 'mass screening' and one must recognize that they have been successful. Neuroblastoma screening at 6 to 7 months of age in Kyoto was estimated to include around 70% of area births [10, 11]. The Japanese have demonstrated that this method aimed at the prevention of advanced disease is effective. In a recent report, they have recorded the follow up of 25 children detected by screening almost half a million infants. Twenty-three — 92% — of these patients were disease free with a medium follow-up of more than three years [12]. In the USA, also, there is a tendency to embark on such a program [13]. Why not in Europe? The economic and emotional impact of advanced neuroblastoma is very high. If there is a possibility to 'prevent' such a devastating disease, why not try to apply it?

1.1.3 Prognostic significance of VMA:HVA ratio

Conflicting results have been reported concerning the correlation of VMA and HVA levels in pretreatment urines and prognosis of neuroblastoma patients.

High initial VMA levels were associated with a poor prognosis in one study [14] whereas in other reports no significant correlation was found between the levels of HVA or VMA and prognosis [15, 16]. An unfavourable outlook has also been shown in children with a high HVA:(VMA+VLA) [17] or HVA:VMA [16] ratio. An HVA:VMA ratio that is greater than unity would indicate a functionally undifferentiated tumour and, consequently, a poorer prognosis with respect to time to progress only, not survival. Finally, in a retrospective study of 336 children with advanced neuroblastoma, neither HVA or VMA levels at diagnosis nor the HVA:VMA ratio had any prognostic value [18].

1.2 Plasma HVA and VMA

Using the mass-fragmentographic method, Gahr and Hunneman determined the plasma levels of HVA and VMA before treatment in 84 children of histologically confirmed neuroblastoma as well as in 15 patients presenting with relapse. The urinary levels of these catecholamine metabolites were also measured at the same time. Their results were recently reported [19]. They showed that the determination of catecholamine metabolites in plasma could be used for diagnosis and monitoring of neuroblastoma patients with at least as much reliability as determination in urine. In a few cases, elevated plasma levels were even found although urine levels were reported as normal. In an earlier study, Krivit and coworkers had established that serum HVA and VMA concentrations were elevated in children with stage IV neuroblastoma and that they tended to parallel urinary levels [20]. Prospective studies should now be undertaken to compare plasma–serum levels and random urine determination of catecholamine metabolite levels. If the results are comparable, the test performed on random urines would be the investigation of choice for neuroblastoma.

2. NEURON-SPECIFIC ENOLASE

Enolase is a glycolytic enzyme which catalyses the conversion of 2-phosphoglycerate to phosphoenolpyruvate. Brain and neuroendocrine tissues contain two forms of enolases, denoted $\alpha\alpha$ and $\gamma\gamma$ enolase to indicate that they are dimers of biochemically and immunologically distinct subunits. A hybrid form ($\alpha\gamma$), with intermediate biochemical and immunological properties, is also present in these tissues. In brain,the $\alpha\alpha$ enolase is confined to glial cells, while the $\gamma\gamma$ form is found in neurons and therefore has been called neuron-specific enolase (NSE). NSE is further found in the amine precursor uptake and decarboxylation (APUD) cells. In addition to the $\alpha\alpha$ enolase, which is found in most cells, and NSE, a third form of enolase ($\beta\beta$) is present in muscle cells.

NSE has been detected in most tumours of neuroectodermal or neuroendocrine origin including neuroblastoma and small cell carcinoma of the lung. Elevated serum NSE levels in patients with these tumours have been reported, as documented for patients with neuroblastoma [21, 22], small cell carcinoma of the lung [23] and pancreatic islet cell carcinoma [24].

The problems posed in the determination of serum NSE levels in suspected or confirmed neuroblastoma patients are those of the marker's specificity and sensitivity of the measuring technique.

More specifically, is serum NSE higher than the norm in all children with neuroblastoma? Does it return to normal levels during remission? Does it increase before a relapse becomes clinically or radiologically detectable?

2.1 Is serum NSE specific of neuroblastoma in paediatric oncology?

Using the Pharmacia NSE double-antibody radioimmunoassay, serum NSE was measured in children with neuroblastoma, retinoblastoma and other malignancies and children with non-malignant diseases attending our department (Fig. 2) [25]. The median NSE value for the children admitted for assessment of a malignancy other than a neuroblastoma or retinoblastoma — 10 μg/l — was not significantly different from the normal values. However, elevated serum NSE was found in one child with ALL (62 μg/l), one with acute monoblastic leukaemia (29 μg/l), one with Wilms' tumour (16.1 μg/l) and one with histiosarcoma (14 μg/l). For the children with retinoblastoma, which, like neuroblastoma, belongs to the 'neurocristopathy', the median value was higher at diagnosis (14.9 μg/l) than during the follow-up period (7.2 μg/l). Finally, for the children being managed for neuroblastoma, the median values were very high — and almost identical — at both diagnosis (68 μg/l) and relapse (50 μg/l), where the median value was almost identical to the normal value (7.6 μg/l) during the follow-up period. This small series suggests that, although high serum NSE levels are suggestive of neuroblastoma, increased NSE levels can be seen in other childhood malignancies. This has been demonstrated in other larger series where raised serum NSE levels have been noted in children with Wilms' tumour,

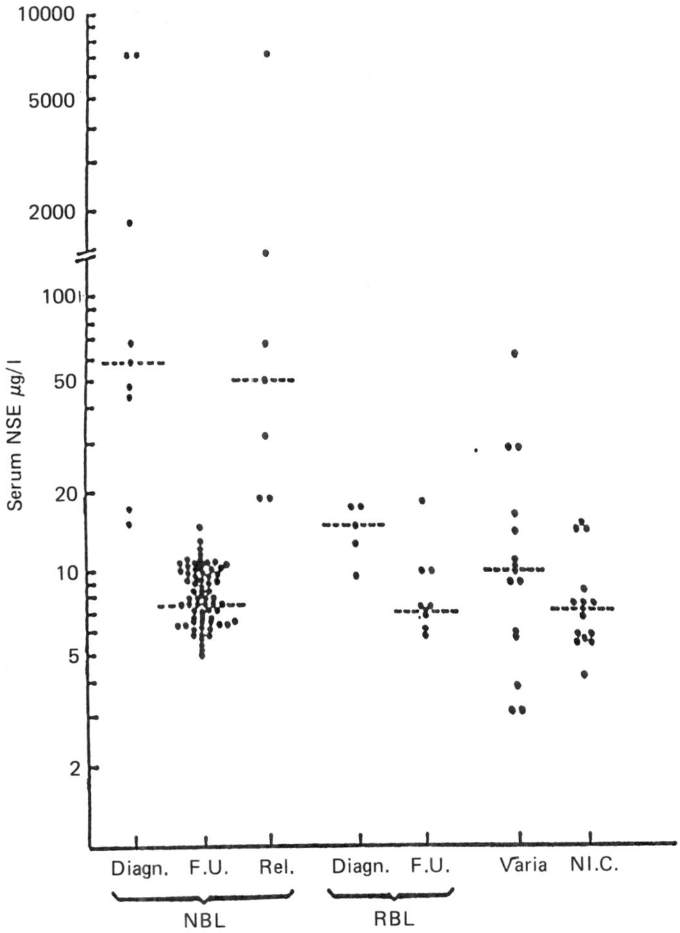

Fig. 2 — Serum NSE specificity. NBL, neuroblastoma; RBL, retinoblastoma; Varia, other malignancies; Nl.C., normal controls; Diagn., at diagnosis; F.U., follow-up; Rel., relapse; (—●—, median value.) (From Ninane [25].)

Ewing's sarcoma, non-Hodgkin lymphoma, soft tissue sarcoma and acute leukaemias [26–28], indicating that caution should be exercised in using this serum marker as a diagnostic test in children with malignancies.

2.2 Is serum NSE useful in the follow-up of children with neuroblastoma?

The serum NSE levels of two patients with advanced neuroblastoma during the course of their disease are shown in Fig. 3 [25]. After two months of chemotherapy, their NSE titres returned to normal, although the primary tumour could still be demonstrated. Still, the gradual increase in the serum NSE levels of one patient preceded both the clinical and the radiological diagnosis of his relapse. The experience of serial measurements in children with neuroblastoma during treatment is limited but it would appear that levels can return to normal early during

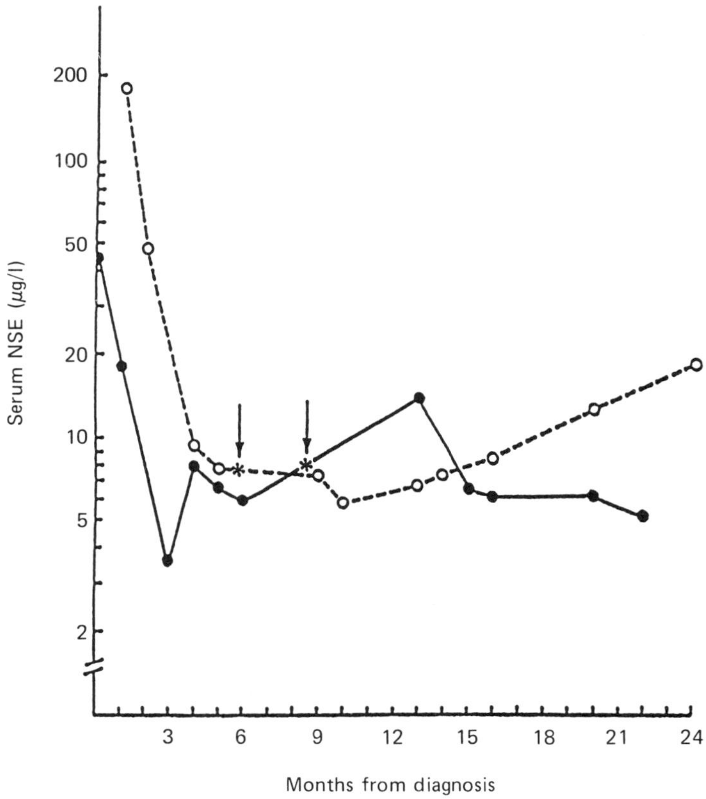

Fig. 3 — Serum NSE sensitivity. Serial measurements of serum NSE in two children with advanced neuroblastoma. *denotes high-dose Melphalan and autologous bone marrow rescue. (From Ninane [25].)

chemotherapy, at a time when there is still clinical and radiological evidence of residual disease. Thus, the test is not particularly sensitive and it remains to be demonstrated that serial NSE measurements are more valuable than serial catecholamine levels in monitoring children with neuroblastoma [29].

2.3 Is serum NSE a useful factor of prognosis in children with neuroblastoma?

Raised serum NSE levels can be found in all stages of neuroblastoma at diagnosis. However, patients with the smallest tumour mass (stages I and II) have the lowest range of serum NSE values whereas patients with advanced disease (stages III and IV) have the highest levels of NSE [27, 28]. In general, a low level predicts a good prognosis and a high level a poor outcome but this is mainly due to the fact that children with localized neuroblastoma present with much lower serum NSE levels than children with advanced disease [27, 28]. Finally, it is interesting to notice that patients with IV-S neuroblastoma have much lower serum NSE levels than children with stage IV neuroblastoma [28]. Although the stage IV-S infants have in general a large tumour burden, this confirms the less aggressive behaviour of this particular form of disseminated neuroblastoma and its better prognosis.

3. FERRITIN

The iron-containing compounds in the body may be conveniently grouped in two categories: those known to serve a metabolic or enzymatic function and those associated with iron storage and transport. The latter category includes the storage compounds ferritin and haemosiderin which are present primarily in the liver and reticuloendothelial cells and in the erythroid precursors of the bone marrow. The protein portion of ferritin, apoferritin, consists of 24 polypeptide chains, with a total molecular weight of 450 000. These 24 subunits form a spherical cluster around variable amounts of hydrated ferric phosphate contained within a central colloidal core. Ferritin contains up to 25% iron by weight and has a molecular weight as high as 900 000, depending on its iron content. There are at least two types of ferritin subunits, and different ratios of the two are believed to account for different electrophoretic patterns of ferritin from various organs and tissues. The liver and spleen contain the most basic isoferritins, whereas the heart contains the most acidic isoferritins. As is the case for most plasma proteins, a high proportion of ferritin is glycosylated during secretion and glycosylated ferritin in serum can bind to concanavilin A (Con A), a plant lectin that binds glycoproteins that contain glucose and/or mannose residues. It has also been observed that ferritins released directly from damaged cells, as in the case of massive hepatic necrosis, do not bind to Con A [30]. Children with advanced neuroblastoma frequently present with an increased level of ferritin in serum and the levels usually decrease during treatment and may return to normal values when the patients are in clinical remission [31].

3.1 Source of increased ferritin in neuroblastoma

Increased amounts of serum ferritin in patients with neuroblastoma can, in theory, be due to tissue damage caused by tumour invasion, to an increase of unused iron associated with anaemia, to a leakage of neuroblastoma cell ferritin during tumour necrosis or to an augmented synthesis of ferritin by neuroblastoma cells and subsequent secretion in plasma.

Evidence that tumour cells are, at least in part, responsible for the elevated ferritins often found in the serum of patients with neuroblastoma has been given by studies of animal models and in children.

Hann and colleagues clearly demonstrated that transplanted human neuroblastoma cells produce human ferritins in the circulation of nude mice, supporting the hypothesis that elevated ferritin levels in patients with neuroblastoma originate, at least in part, from their tumours [32]. The same group [33] then showed that much of the increased ferritin in sera of children with neuroblastoma was bound to Con A, indicating that ferritin was glycosylated. Since it was demonstrated earlier that glycosylated ferritin is present in the serum through the secretion process [30], this could mean that raised levels of serum ferritin in children with neuroblastoma are the result of increased synthesis followed by secretion of the molecule in plasma.

3.2 Prognostic significance of serum ferritin in patients with neuroblastoma

Ferritin is not frequently elevated in sera from children with stage I and II neuroblastomas but is abnormally raised in some patients with stage III and IV diseases (Table 1) [34]. Analysis of event-free survival for children with stage III and

Table 1 — Serum ferritin and stage of neuroblastoma (adapted from Hann *et al.* [34])

Stage	Numbers of patients			% Raised
	Total	Raised Ferritin	Normal Ferritin	
I	7	0	7	0
II	21	4	17	19
III	38	14	24	37
IV	175	94	81	54

IV neuroblastomas indicates that raised ferritin was at diagnosis associated with a significantly poorer prognosis than normal ferritin and that this correlation is independent of stage and age at diagnosis [34]. For stage III patients in particular, those with normal ferritin have a survival rate of 75% at two years whereas those with elevated ferritin have a survival rate of only 12% at two years from diagnosis [34]. Recently, known prognostic factors in neuroblastoma were analysed in 124 children with neuroblastoma diagnosed and treated at the Children's Hospital of Philadelphia [35] in order to determine which were independent and which were most useful in predicting outcome. When recursive partitioning was performed, the analysis produced a tree which was first split on normal vs. elevated serum ferritin and was further defined by splits based on age and stage of disease. This analysis produced three primary groups of children with different prognoses: good (normal ferritin, age less than two years; two-year survival of 93%), intermediate (normal ferritin, age two years or older; two-year survival of 58%) and poor (raised ferritin; two-year survival of 19%) (Fig. 4) [35].

4. GANGLIOSIDES

Gangliosides, sialic-acid-containing glycosphingolipids, are mainly detected in the cell surface membrane. The highest concentrations of gangliosides are found in brain tissue. However, they are present in all tissues, including tumours. These membrane-bound glycolipids are shed or released *in vitro* by a variety of cells, particularly tumour cells [36] and high concentrations of gangliosides have been demonstrated in the plasma of tumour-bearing animals [37]. It now appears that these markers are present in both the tumours and the plasma of most children with neuroblastoma.

4.1 Circulating gangliosides in neuroblastoma patients

Using a quantitative competitive enzyme-linked immunosorbent assay, Schulz and colleagues [38] studied the disialoganglioside G_{D2} in the serum of children with neuroblastoma and other solid tumours.

In children with active neuroblastoma, 21 of 23 exhibited raised G_{D2} levels in serum. The two children with lower levels had stage I and II disease. Six children, who after treatment were considered disease free, showed normal levels of G_{D2} in

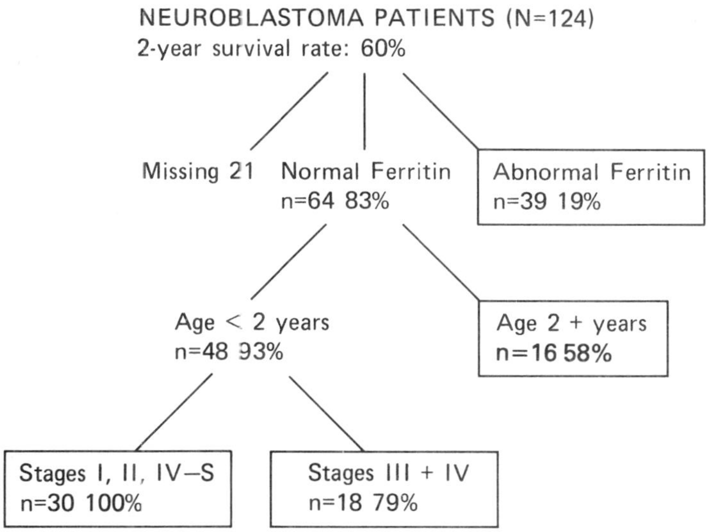

Fig. 4 — Prognostic factor of ferritin levels in children with neuroblastoma. Arborization is made until there is no additional factor affecting the prognosis. *, survival rate at 2 years from diagnosis. (From Evans *et al.* [35].)

their serum. Among the 23 children with other malignancies, only 2 showed elevated G_{D2} levels in their serum. One child had a Wilms' tumour and the other an osteogenic sarcoma. Two other patients with Wilms' tumour as well as one other child with osteogenic sarcoma had normal levels of G_{D2}. Finally, in one 16-month old child with neuroblastoma, these authors were able to follow the serum level of G_{D2} during the clinical course of the disease and showed a remarkable correlation between the decreased levels of the ganglioside and the regression of tumour size.

Other investigators showed that the circulating concentration of G_{D2} ganglioside in patients with neuroblastoma reveals that important shedding of this ganglioside is associated with the presence of tumour. Ladisch and Wu, in a preliminary communication [39], demonstrated that G_{D2} is a major ganglioside of neuroblastoma tumour tissue and was present in the plasma of five patients with widespread neuroblastoma. In contrast, the ganglioside was not detected in plasma samples of six patients in complete remission or in plasma samples of 17 healthy subjects. The same authors then extended their studies to more patients and reported on 32 children with neuroblastoma [40]. Using direct thin-layer chromatographic analysis, they studied the G_{D2} concentrations in plasma of children at diagnosis and during the course of their disease. Among the 32 neuroblastoma patients in all clinical stages evaluated before treatment, 27 (84%) showed elevated plasma concentrations of the disialoganglioside G_{D2}, the mean level being more than 50 times the normal plasma G_{D2} concentration. Moreover, circulating G_{D2} was not detected in the plasma of children with ganglioneuroblastoma or ganglioneuroma, indicating an association of the shedding of this ganglioside with undifferentiated neuroblastoma only.

Finally, in their series, the sequential determination of circulating G_{D2} revealed that plasma levels diminished in children responding to therapy and reappeared in patients in relapse.

4.2 Ganglioside composition of neuroblastomas: a prognostic factor?

A preliminary study of the ganglioside composition of six neuroblastomas suggested that the lack of G_{T1b} might indicate a poor prognosis [41]. Since that study was reported, the ganglioside composition of 47 additional neuroblastomas was studied by the same investigators who have recently published their findings about the whole series of 53 tumours [42]. The presence of G_{D2} in 45 of the tumour samples correlates well with the fact that the serum G_{D2} may serve as a marker in children with neuroblastoma (see above) [38, 40] and the lack of detectable G_{D2} in tumour tissues from eight patients of that series may explain the failure of Schulz and colleagues to detect raised levels of G_{D2} in the serum from 2 of the 23 children they studied (see above) [38]. Also, G_{D2} was absent in four ganglioneuroma tumour samples, suggesting — as from the serum data (see above) [40] — that the presence of G_{D2} may reflect the presence of immature neurons. Of most importance, however, is the fact that tumours lacking G_{T1b} seem to indicate a poor prognosis. Indeed, six of the seven children with absence of G_{T1b} in their neuroblastoma died of their disease. This finding is even more striking for the subset of 20 children with mediastinal neuroblastoma. Tumours from patients with thoracic primaries were found to contain more complex gangliosides of the b series — G_{D1b} and G_{T1b} — and fewer monosialogangliosides, suggesting a more differentiated cellular composition [42, 43]. Only one child of the 20 with mediastinal primary lacked G_{T1b} in his tumour and died of disease. These very interesting data suggest that the better prognosis universally reported for children with thoracic neuroblastoma, as compared with other sites, is probably due to a biological difference within the membrane of the tumour cells.

4.3 Gangliosides as a target of antineuroblastoma therapy?

The fact that disialoganglioside G_{D2} is present in the membrane of most neuroblastoma cells may lead to the possibility of 'targeting' therapy. This has been successfully performed, at least in an animal model. A murine monoclonal antibody directed against G_{D2} was labelled with ^{131}I and injected into nude mice bearing human neuroblastoma xenografts [44]. The tumours that received more than 4200 cGy were completely ablated without recurrence and with acceptable toxicity for the hosts. These preliminary encouraging results deserve of course confirmation before this technique is applied in children with neuroblastoma.

5. CONCLUSIONS

The ideal neuroblastoma marker is a molecule of neuroblastoma cell origin, released in the circulation and/or in the urine of the patient in amounts easily detectable and proportional to the stage of the disease. Moreover, the molecule should not be present in substantial concentrations in the circulation and/or urine of children in remission or in the circulation and/or urine of children with other diseases. Not all the above criteria for an ideal neuroblastoma marker are met by catecholamines, NSE, ferritin and gangliosides taken individually. In institutions with good clinical research facilities, these four markers should ideally be examined at the same time.

However, random samples of urine for sequential determination of HVA and VMA probably constitute the best test if one considers its sensitivity and its specificity on the one hand and — above all — the comfort of the child on the other hand.

REFERENCES

[1] Greenberg, R. E. & Gardner, L. I. (1959). New diagnosis test for neural tumors of infancy. Increased urinary excretion of 3-methoxy-4-hydroxy-mandelic acid and norepinephrine in a ganglioneuroma with chronic diarrhea. *Pediatrics* **24** 683–684

[2] Stickler, G. B., Hallenbeck, G. A. & Flock, E. V. (1959). Ganglioneuroblastoma associated with chronic diarrhoea and increased excretion of catecholamines. *Proc. Staff Meet. Mayo Clin.* **34** 548–549

[3] von Studnitz, W. (1961). Occurrence, isolation and identification of 3-methoxy-4-hydroxy phenylalanine. *Clin. Chem. Acta* **6** 525–530

[4] Armstrong, M. D., McMillan, A. & Shaw, K. (1957). 3-methoxy-4-hydroxy-D-mandelic acid, a urinary metabolite of norepinephrine. *Biochem. Biophys. Acta* **25** 422–423

[5] Soldin, S. J. & Hill, J. G. (1980). Simultaneous liquid-chromatographic analysis for 4-hydroxy-3-methoxymandelic acid and 4-hydroxy-3-methoxyphenylacetic acid in urine. *Clin. Chem.* **26** 291–294

[6] Tuchman, M., Crippin, P. J. & Krivit, W. (1983). Capillary gas chromatographic determination of urinary homovanillic acid and vanillylmandelic acid. *Clin. Chem.* **29** 828–831

[7] Tuchman, M., Morris, L., Ramnaraine, M. *et al.* (1985). Value of random urinary homovanillic acid and vanillymandelic acid levels in the diagnosis and management of patients with neuroblastoma: comparison with 24-hour urine collections. *Pediatrics* **75** 324–328

[8] Tuchman, M., Ramnaraine, M., Woods, W. & Krivit, W. (1987). Three years of experience with random urinary homovanillic and vanillylmandelic acid levels in the diagnosis of neuroblastoma. *Pediatrics* **79** 203–205

[9] Pritchard, J., Kiely, E., Rogers, D. W. *et al.* (1987). Long-term survival after advanced neuroblastoma. *N. Engl. J. Med.* **317** 1026–1027 (letter)

[10] Sawada, T., Todo, S., Fujita, K. *et al.* (1984). Neuroblastoma, mass screening for early detection and its prognosis. *Cancer* **53** 2731–2735

[11] Sawada, T., Nakata, T., Tagasugi, N. *et al.* (1984). Mass screening for neuroblastoma in infants in Japan. *Lancet* **2** 271–273

[12] Sawada, T. (1986). Outcome of 25 neuroblastoma revealed by screening in Japan. *Lancet* **1** 377 (letter)

[13] Woods, G. W. & Tuchman, M. (1987). Neuroblastoma: the case for screening infants in North America. *Pediatrics* **79** 869–873

[14] Gitlow, S. E., Dziedzig, L. B., Strauss, L. *et al.* (1973). Biochemical and histologic determinants in the prognosis of neuroblastoma. *Cancer* **32** 898–905

[15] Labrosse, E. M., Comay, E., Bohuan, C. *et al.* (1976). Catecholamine metabolism in neuroblastoma. *J. Natl. Cancer Inst.* **57** 633–638

[16] Siegel, S. E., Laug, W. E., Harlow, P. J. *et al.* (1980). Patterns of urinary

catecholamine metabolite excretion in neuroblastoma. In: A. E. Evans (ed.) *Advances in Neuroblastoma Research,* Raven Press, New York, pp. 25–32

[17] Voûte, P. A., Van Putten, W. J. & Burgers, J. M. (1975). Tumors of the sympathetic nervous system. In: H. Bloom, J. Lemerle, M. Nerhardt & P. Voûte (eds.) *Cancer in Children, Clinical Management,* Springer Verlag, New York, pp. 138–148

[18] Ninane, J., Vangyseghem, S., André, F. *et al.* (1986). Long term survivors of advanced neuroblastoma: factors affecting prognosis. An ENSG study (abstract) *International Society of Pediatric Oncology, XVIII Meeting, Belgrade, Yugoslavia, September 15–20*

[19] Gahr, M. & Hunneman, D. H. (1987). The value of determination of homovanillic and vanillylmandelic acids in plasma for the diagnosis and follow-up of neuroblastoma in children.*Eur. J. Pediatr.* **146** 489–493

[20] Krivit, W., Mirkin, B. L., Freier, E. *et al.* (1980). Serum catecholamine metabolites in stage IV neuroblastoma. In: A. E. Evans (ed.) *Advances in Neuroblastoma Research,* Raven Press, New York, pp. 33–42

[21] Ishiguro, Y., Kato, K., Shimizu, A. *et al.* (1982). High levels of immunoreactive nervous system-specific enolase in sera of patients with neuroblastoma. *Clin. Chem. Acta* **121** 173–180

[22] Zeltzer, P. M., Marangos, P. J., Parma, A. M. *et al.* (1983). Raised neuron-specific enolase in serum of children with metastasic neuroblastoma. *Lancet* **2** 361–363

[23] Pahlman, S., Esschert, T., Bergh, J. *et al.* (1984). Neuron-specific enolase as a marker for neuroblastoma and small cell carcinoma of the lung. *Tumour Biol.* **452** 245–252

[24] Prinz, R. A. & Marangos, P. J. (1983). Serum neuron-specific enolase: a serum marker for non-functioning pancreatic islet cell carcinoma. *Am J. Surg.* **145** 77–81

[25] Ninane, J. (1987). Childhood neuroblastoma. Diagnostic and therapeutic strategy. *Thesis.* University of Louvain, Belgium.

[26] Pritchard, J., Cooper, E. H., Hamilton, S. *et al.* (1987). Serum neuron-specific enolase may be raised in children with Wilms' tumour. *Lancet* **1** 110 (letter)

[27] Cooper, E. H., Pritchard, J., Bailey, C. C. & Ninane, J. (1987). Serum neuron-specific enolase in childrens' cancer. *Br. J. Cancer* **56** 65–67

[28] Zeltzer, P. M., Marangos, P. J., Evans, A. E. *et al.* (1986). Serum neuron-specific enolase in children with neuroblastoma. Relationship to stage and disease course. *Cancer* **57** 1230–1234

[29] Hashimoto, K., Gotoh, Y.-I. & Tada, K. (1986). Serum neuron-specific enolase as a marker useful for monitoring the effectiveness of therapy in patients with neuroblastoma — as compared with urinary catecholamines metabolites. *Tohoku J. Exp. Med.* **149** 25–30

[30] Worwood, M., Cragg, S. J., Wagstaff, M. *et al.* (1979). Binding of human serum ferritin to concanavilin A. *Clin. Sci.* **56** 83–87

[31] Hann, H. L., Levy, H. M. & Evans, A. E. (1980). Serum ferritin as a guide to therapy in neuroblastoma. *Cancer Res.* **40** 1411–1413

[32] Hann, H. L., Stahlhut, M. W. & Millman, I. (1984). Human ferritins present in the sera of nude mice transplanted with human neuroblastoma or hepatocellu-

lar carcinoma. *Cancer Res.* **44** 3898–3901

[33] Hann, H. L., Stahlhut, M. W. & Evans, A. E. (1986). Source of increased ferritin in neuroblastoma: studies with concanavilin A–sepharose binding. *J. Natl. Cancer Inst.* **76** 1031–1033

[34] Hann, H. L., Evans, A. E., Siegel, S. E. *et al.* (1985). Prognostic importance of serum ferritin in patients with stages III and IV neuroblastoma: the children's Cancer Study Group experience. *Cancer Res.* **45** 2843–2848

[35] Evans, A. E., D'Angio, G. J., Propert, K. *et al.* (1987). Prognostic factors in neuroblastoma. *Cancer* **59** 1853–1859

[36] Black, P. H. (1980). Shedding from the cell surface of normal and cancer cells. *Adv. Cancer Res.* **32** 75–199

[37] Lengle, E. E. (1979). Increased levels of lipid-bound sialic acid in thymic lymphocytes and plasma of leukemic AKR/J mice. *J. Natl. Cancer Inst.* **62** 1565–1567

[38] Schulz, G., Cheresh, D. A., Varki, N. M. *et al.* (1984). Detection of ganglioside G_{D2} in tumor tissues and sera of neuroblastoma patients. *Cancer Res.* **44** 5914–5920

[39] Ladisch, S. & Wu, Z. L. (1985). Detection of a tumour-associated ganglioside in plasma of patients with neuroblastoma. *Lancet* **1** 136–139

[40] Ladisch, S., Wu, Z. L., Feig, S., *et al.* (1987). Shedding of G_{D2} ganglioside by human neuroblastoma. *Int. J. Cancer* **39** 73–76

[41] Shochat, S. J., Abt, A. B. & Schengrund, C.-L. (1977). VCN-releasable sialic acid and gangliosides in human neuroblastomas. *J. Pediatr. Surg.* **12** 413–418

[42] Schengrund, C.-L., Repman, M. A. & Schochat, S. (1985). Ganglioside composition of human neuroblastomas. Correlation with prognosis. A pediatric oncology group study. *Cancer* **56** 2640–2646

[43] Schochat, S., Corbelletta, N., Repman, M. & Schengrund, C.-L. (1987). A biochemical analysis of thoracic neuroblastomas: a pediatric oncology group study. *J. Pediatr Surg.* **22** 660–664

[44] Cheung, N.-K., Landmeier, B., Neely, J. *et al.* (1986). Complete tumor ablation with iodine 131-radiolabeled disialoganglioside G_{D2}-specific monoclonal antibody against tumour neuroblastoma xenografted in nude mice. *J. Natl. Cancer Inst.* **77** 739–745

3

Molecular genetics of human neuroblastoma

M. Schwab
Institut für Experimentelle Pathologie, Deutsches Krebsforschungszentrum, D–6900 Heidelberg, FRG

1. INTRODUCTION

Three types of chromosomal abnormalities are frequently associated with human neuroblastoma: (1) deletions of the short arm of chromosome 1; (2) 'double minutes' (DMs); (3) 'homogeneously staining chromosomal regions' (HSRs). The significance of chromosome 1 deletion is still unclear, owing to lack of knowledge about the genetic information deleted. In contrast, the role of DMs and HSRs has come to a closer understanding. Both chromosomal abnormalities contain amplified cellular DNA. By serendipitous analyses a gene, N-*myc*, has been identified that is capable of contributing to control of cellular growth. N-*myc* is a member of the cellular growth control genes, generally referred to as cellular oncogenes. The frequent association of N-*myc* amplification with higher malignant forms of neuroblastoma make it likely that enhanced expression consequent to amplification is a factor conferring growth properties on the host cell.

2. CHROMOSOME 1 DELETIONS

Deletions of chromosome 1 were first described in 1975 [7]. Even though the breakpoints of the deletion were found to vary, the portion of the chromosome distal to band p32 seems to be most consistently deleted (Fig. 1). In all cases, the deletions involve only one chromosome. From cytogenetic analyses the portion deleted appears to be lost from the genome, which means that the cells are monosomic for this genetic material

At this point, the nature of the genetic material deleted and its significance to tumorigenesis can only be the subject of speculation. There is a good possibility that the deletion involves genetic information essential for normal differentiation of certain neutral cells. Loss could result in abnormal differentiation and could be a factor contributing to tumorigenesis. In a similar way lack of genetic information

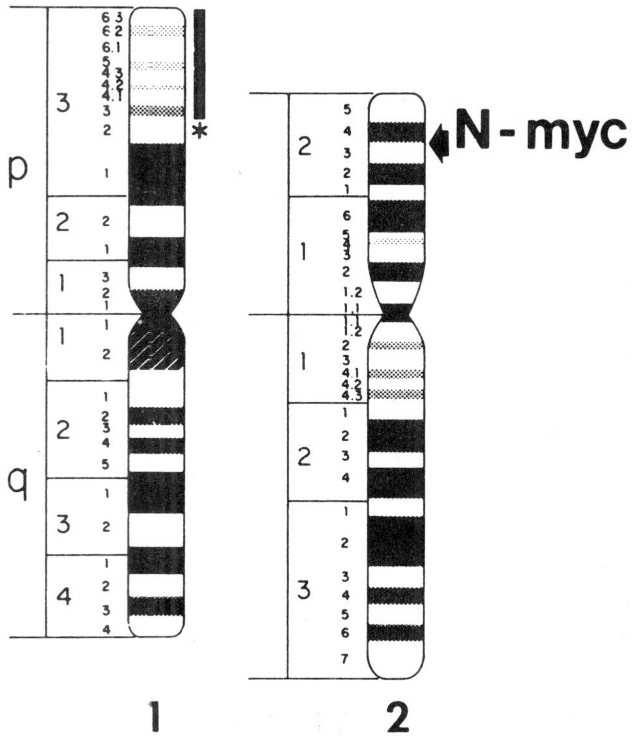

Fig. 1 — Genes involved in human neuroblastoma. Loss of genetic material of chromosome 1 and amplification of genes of chromosome 2 seem to contribute in many cases to neuroblastoma.

identified by cytogenetic analysis in specific regions of other chromosomes seems to contribute to other types of tumours, in particular Wilm's tumour, retinoblastoma, lung cancer and certain forms of colon cancer (for a review see [2]). The general idea is that the presence of this genetic information supresses tumorigenesis and its lack allows tumours to develop. Genes behaving as suppressors of tumorigenesis have been termed 'tumour-suppressor' genes, although their functions and the mechanisms by which they act are obscure as yet.

3. DMs AND HSRs

The most conspicuous chromosomal abnormality of neuroblastoma cells are the DMs. Originally discovered as early as 1965 in cells of direct preparations of a malignant neuroblastoma [1], DMs were subsequently found in nearly all types of human tumours [3]. DMs seem to be unique to malignant or transformed cells. Origin, genetic information and significance to tumorigenesis have been a matter of speculation for many years [4,5]. HSR regions were discovered in 1973 [6] and were found to be present in a variety of types of tumours. In spite of the ubiquitous occurrence of DMs and HSRs in human and animal tumours, human neuroblastoma appears to be the tumour type most frequently showing these chromosomal abnormalities.

4. AMPLIFICATION OF DNA

Experimental systems had unveiled in several cases DMs and HSRs as cytogenetic manifestations of amplified cellular DNA. In particular, cells resistant to therapeutic drugs, such as methotrexate, were shown to carry amplified copies of the gene dihydrofolate-reductase (see [8] for review). Because in many cases untreated neuroblastoma cells carry DMs and HSRs, acquired drug resistance is an unlikely explanation for the presence of amplified DNA.

Two molecular approaches have been used to define the significance of the amplified DNA and to identify functional genes within. First, by differential hybridization procedures a panel of amplified DNA sequences was isolated from neuroblastoma cell line IMR-32 and shown to be derived from the HSR localized on chromosome 1 [9]. The genetic complexity of the HSR was estimated to be approximately 3000 kilobase pairs. Interestingly, the amplified sequences were shown to be derived from chromosome 2, by analysing chromosomes of normal lymphocytes. Furthermore, in IMR-32 cells, sequences amplified within the HSR on chromosome 1 could be shown to be present in what appears to be a single copy on chromosome 2. Apparently the strategy by which neuroblasts amplify cellular DNA involves extra replication of portions of chromosome 2p followed by generation of extrachromosomal DNA, perhaps as DMs, which in turn can become more or less randomly integrated at different chromosomal positions. Interestingly, HSR regions have so far been found in different neuroblastomas on over 20 different chromosomes [10].

The second approach involved surveys of human neuroblastoma cells for amplification of proto-oncogenes (see [11,12] for review). Conditions of reduced stringency allowed the identification of an amplified gene, N-*myc*, closely related to the proto-oncogene c-*myc* [13,14].

Analysis of DNA of a series of different neuroblastoma cell lines with random probes [15] revealed that the amplified DNA is heterogeneous [16]. DNA amplified in cells from one neuroblastoma may not be amplified in others. N-*myc* seems to be localized in the core region of the amplified unit and is consistently amplified [17] as if a selective force is favouring retention of N-*myc*. At this point all the experimental evidence indicates N-*myc* to be the selective growth control gene responsible for the maintenance of the amplified unit.

5. THE N-*myc* GENE

N-*myc* is highly related in structure and nucleotid sequence to the proto-oncogene c-*myc*, which is the authentic cellular homologue of the oncogene c-*myc* of the chicken retrovirus MH29. N-*myc* is but one member of a multigene family referred to as *myc*-box genes [18]. Another member, L-*myc*, has been found frequently amplified in human small cell lung cancer cells [19,20]. N-*myc* and L-*myc* may be members of a family of *myc*- related genes that are evolutionarily conserved among vertebrates [18]. The human *myc* genes identified to date are dispersed on different chromosomes: c-*myc* is localised at 8q24–ter [21], N-*myc* at 2p23–24 [22], and L-*myc* at 1p32 [19].

Amplification of N-*myc* has been found in neuroblastoma cell lines and in tumours derived directly from patients not subjected to chemo- or radiotherapy (Fig. 2; reviewed in [12]). DMs and HSRs, the presence of which originally

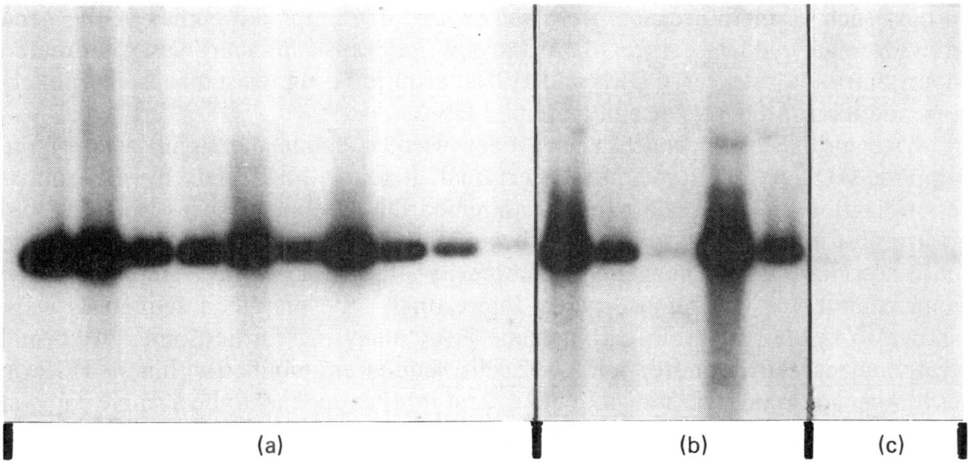

Fig. 2 — Amplification of N-*myc* in neuroblastomas: (a) cell lines, (b) tumours; (c) normal human cells.

stimulated the studies of neuroblastoma, are the sites of the amplified N-*myc* [13,14]. Amplification of N-*myc* has also been found in cell lines derived from small cell lung cancers [23], from a few retinoblastoma tumours and cell lines [24,25] and from one astrocytoma [26].

N-*myc*, like c-*myc*, consists of three exons, interrupted by two intervening sequences (Fig. 3 [27,28]). Exons 2 and 3 have regions of high similarity to the c-*myc* gene. In contrast, exon 1 does not show obvious similarity of the nucleotide sequence between N-*myc* and c-*myc*. The coding region is confined to exons 2 and 3. The mature N-*myc* mRNA is approximately 3.0 kb in length and is translated into a protein with apparent molecular weight of 67 kilodalton. The N-*myc* protein is localized predominantly within the nucleus of the cell, and binds to DNA under experimental conditions [29,30].

6. THE ONCOGENIC POTENTIAL OF N-*myc*

The oncogenic potential of N-*myc* has been addressed in various cell systems, mainly derived from rat. The basic principle has been that expression vectors containing N-*myc* were introduced into test cells. Subsequently the behaviour of the cells has been analysed with respect to various parameters, such as establishment of primary cells in culture, growth in soft agar and under reduced serum conditions, and tumorigenicity. The N-*myc* expression vectors pMP-34.1^{K} and pMP-34.1^{N} contain the U3 region of long terminal repeat (LTR) of Moloney murine leukaemia virus (MoMLV) covalently linked to the N-*myc* gene derived from neuroblastoma line Kelly (pMP-34.1^{K}) and from leukocytes of a normal individual (pMP-34.1^{N}). A derivative of

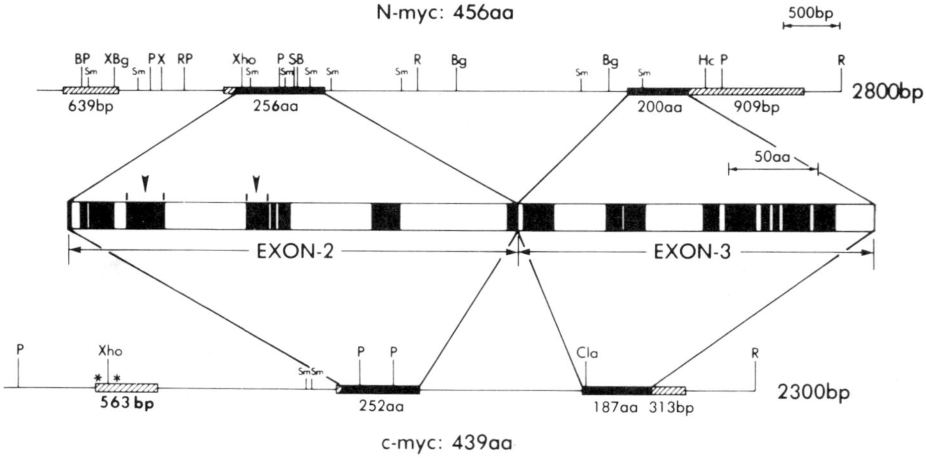

Fig. 3 — Structural comparison between human N-*myc* and c-*myc*. The top and bottom drawings display the topography of the N-*myc* and c-*myc* genes respectively. Solid areas present coding regions, hatched areas non-coding portions, and lines intervening sequences and flanking DNA (for more detailed information and for restriction endonuclease sites in N-*myc* and c-*myc* see Stanton *et al.* [27]. (1983)). Asterisks over non-coding exon 1 in c-*myc* indicate the two promoter sites. N-*myc* contains multiple initiation sites (at least 14), causing a variation in the size of the exon (between roughly 450 and 600 base pairs). The numbers at the extreme right refer to the average size of the N-*myc* and c-*myc* mRNA without considering the poly(A)-tail. The centre drawing presents a comparison of the deduced amino acid sequences of N-*myc* and c-*myc*. Black areas indicate regions where the amino acid homology exceeds 70%. Arrowheads over top of two black areas in exon 2 indicate the positions of the *myc*-boxes in which amino acid homology is greater than 90%.

pMP-34.1^{K} contains a frameshift mutation within the first coding exon (pMP-34.1^{K} ΔXho), rendering the expression vector unable to encode a normal N-*myc* protein (the vectors are described in [31]).

During these experiments N-*myc* has been shown to establish low passage rat cells in long term culture [32], to convert established rat cells (Rat-1 cells) to tumorigenesis [33] and to assist mutationally activated c-Ha-*ras*1 in tumorigenic conversion of low passage rat embryo cells [31].

Altogether, these studies have shown that enhanced expression of N-*myc*, similar to that in neuroblastoma cells carrying 150-fold amplification, is an efficient factor in controlling cellular growth and in conferring tumorigenic properties upon host cells. We assume that enhanced expression consequent to amplification contributes to the malignant phenotype of the neuroblastoma cell.

7. NORMAL FUNCTIONS OF N-*myc*

Normal expression of N-*myc* has been found generally in cells with a low degree of differentiation, particularly in neuroblasts [34–36], in normal and transformed retinoblasts [37], and in normal cells of kidney as well as in nephroblastoma (Wilm's tumour) cells [38]. Particularly high expression, equivalent to that in neuroblastoma cells carrying 150-fold amplified N-*myc*, is present in normal foetal human brain [39]. These observations sustain the suspicion that expression of N-*myc* such as in retinoblastoma cell lines and Wilm's tumours that do not carry amplification is merely a reflection of the state of differentiation these tumour cells might have retained. Expression of N-*myc* without amplification, therefore, is probably in most cases a normal feature of certain undifferentiated cells. One should be cautious, therefore, in relating expression alone of N-*myc*, or any other gene, causally to the neoplastic phenotype of the cell.

N-*myc*, like L-*myc*, is subjected to a strict temporal and spatial expression pattern, as shown by comparison of foetal and adult human brain cells [39] and by analyses of tissues from different stages of the foetal and the developing mouse embryo [34,36], and more detailed information should soon be available by *in situ* hybridization (Karen Downs, personal communication). These results suggest that the *myc*-box genes, either alone or in combination with each other, may play an important role during mammalian development. The c-*myc* gene, in contrast, is virtually not subject to variation in the overall expression during embryonic development. These findings are parallelled by studies of human tumour cells showing almost invariably expression of c-*myc* [40] but, depending on their derivation of embryonic cell lineage, rarely N-*myc* [36]. Altogether, the *myc*-box genes and c-*myc*, in spite of their structural relationship, may have distinctive, different functions. The c-*myc* gene may play a more 'basic' role, whereas N-*myc* and L-*myc* presumably have more specialized functions related to regulation of cellular differentiation.

Specific functions of *myc*-box genes in cell differentiation are also indicated by the specificity at which N-*myc* and c-*myc* are amplified in tumour cells: neuroblastomas have so far exclusively produced N-*myc* amplification, and L-*myc* has been found amplified only in small cell lung cancers. It is possible that the high transcriptional activity during early stages of differentiation favours amplification. The restriction of the expression to certain cell types suggests that N-*myc* is highly regulated and may contribute to specific differentiation pathways. Deregulation, such as the result of amplification, could disrupt the intrinsic control of expression and contribute to the neoplastic phenotype. It is possible that the cellular mechanism evolved to regulate expression of a single copy of N-*myc* is incapable of controlling efficiently expression of multiple gene copies. Strong extrinsic stimuli, such as retinoic acid, are capable, however, of inducing a dramatic decrease in the steady level of N-*myc* mRNA in neuroblastoma cells even when carrying a high degree of amplification [41]. The decrease of the level of N-*myc* mRNA is followed by morphological differentiation of neuroblastoma cells. These studies indicate that regulation of expression of amplified N-*myc* does respond to differentiation-inducing signals. Studies of neuroblastoma tumours in which N-*myc* is amplified have, by *in situ* hybridization, provided evidence for high N-*myc* expression in undifferentiated neuroblasts and for low expression in differentiated ganglion cells [35]. It is tempting to speculate that high, deregulated expression of N-*myc* results in a block of differentiation of neuroblasts to ganglion cells.

8. N-*myc* AND STAGE OF NEUROBLASTOMA

To determine the stage of tumour progression at which amplifications are first detectable, several groups have examined neuroblastomas which have been classified on the basis of various pathological and clinical criteria into Evans stages I–IV, with stage IV being the most advanced. In studies of more than 250 tumours, nearly all of the amplifications detected were present in the more advanced tumours (stages III and IV [42,43]). The estimated progression-free survival over a period of 18 months for standardized therapy was 70% for patients whose tumours lacked amplification and dropped to 30% in cases with 3–10 copies and to 5% in cases with more than 10 copies. It is conceivable that N-*myc* copy number may eventually turn out to be a useful marker for assessing prognosis of neuroblastoma and for devising specific therapeutic regimes.

9. SYNTHESIS

Experimental carcinogenesis studies, as well as clinical evidence, suggest that the development of a malignant tumour is a gradual evolutionary process during which tumour cells progressively acquire permanent, qualitatively different characteristics [44]. Genetic instability of tumour cells has been found to be greatly enhanced over that of normal cells [45], and amplification of DNA may be one of the mechanisms which leads to the emergence of clonal populations with increasingly malignant properties. There is now good experimental evidence that gene amplification occurs in tumorigenic cells at a higher rate than in non-tumorigenic cells [46].

The basal rate of spontaneous amplification of a given genetic locus may be as high as 10^{-3} events per cell generation. The rate at which amplification takes place can be increased severalfold by various extrinsic agents, including metabolic inhibitors, tumour promoters, and carcinogens. The persistence of amplified DNA suggests that there is a selective pressure for their retention. The nature of the selective mechanisms which maintain amplification of proto-oncogenes is at present unknown. A simple but not unlikely explanation could be that the enhanced expression of the amplified proto-oncogene confers a growth advantage upon the host cells within a specific tissue architecture. Amplification of genes could allow the host cells to escape growth control, to become mobile and invasive, or to escape immune surveillance.

The role of amplification of *myc* sequences can also be examined in the light of the multistage nature of tumorigenesis, which often involves the successive steps of initiation and progression. The tight correlation of amplified N-*myc* with advanced disease stages is best explained by assuming that it contributes to malignant progression; however, it is unclear whether this amplification correlates with early or with late phases of progression. Tumour progression, in the sense of Foulds [44], is independent of tumour growth. Staging of neuroblastomas is merely based upon the degree to which the tumour extends beyond the organ or tissue of origin and does not consider the qualitative differences in the tumour cells themselves at early and late phases of progression. It is therefore possible that a particular stage II tumour, for instance, is in a late phase of progression, while a stage III tumour is still in an earlier phase.

Amplification appears to show some specificity in that certain tissues tend to contain a specific amplified proto-oncogene. Analyses of neuroblastomas have revealed amplification only of N-*myc*, Table 1, although N-*myc* and c-*myc* do not differ detectably in their capacity to contribute to the neoplastic transformation of normal rodent cells in tissue culture. L-*myc* has so far been encountered exclusively

Table 1 — Amplification of *myc* genes in different human cancers

		Incidence of cells with amplification of		
		N-*myc*	L-*myc*	c-*myc*
Neuroblastoma	Tumour stage I	0/13	0	0
	Tumour stage II	2/24	0	0
	Tumour stage III	14/43	0	0
	Tumour stage IV	32/45	0	0
	Tumour stage IV–S	0/5	0	0
	Cell lines	22/27	0	0
Retinoblastoma	Tumour	3/27	0	0
	Cell lines	2/16	0	0
Small cell lung carcinoma	Tumours	3	1	0
	Cell lines (classical)	4	4	0
	Cell lines (variant)	1	0	5
Cervical carcinoma	Tumours	0	0	8/12

in small cell lung carcinomas. It remains to be seen whether this specificity is due to preferential amplification at the N-*myc* or L-*myc* locus or whether the particular environment surrounding the host cells selects for amplification of these genes. Although the correlation of N-*myc* amplification with advanced stage of neuroblastoma is striking, major questions remain open. What mechanisms lead to progression of neuroblastomas lacking N-*myc* amplification? May other genes become amplified in these cases? Amplification of other genes seems to be the case in cell line SK-N-MC, derived from a human neuroblastoma. These cells display DMs, but carry only what appears to be single copy of N-*myc*. It is also possible that alternative mechanisms unrelated to gene amplification and not involving N-*myc* contribute to progression. Eventually, staging of neuroblastoma may be only partially related to, or may have nothing to do with the biological process of tumour progression. Primitive neuroectodermal tumours are quite difficult to classify (see [47]). It is possible that tumours classified at the time of presentation actually differ in their cellular derivation, and it is conceivable that, for instance, stage IV tumours with amplification of N-*myc* carry the amplified gene already at early phases of development. In other words, neuroectodermal tumours with amplified N-*myc* could well represent a particular class.

10 FUTURE PERSPECTIVES

Cytogenetic studies of human cancer cells have uncovered the presence of chromosomal abnormalities diagnostic of amplified DNA and have provided an entrance point for molecular biological studies of various human cancers. Amplification of proto-oncogenes is a frequent correlate of malignant progression in some naturally occurring tumours and appears to be a late event unrelated to initiation. These studies have brought attention to a new class of cellular genes related to c-*myc* in very distinct, conserved regions. These *myc*-box genes appear to play an important role during development and cellular differentiation, and their amplification may contribute to progression of tumours derived from embryonic cell lineages in which the *myc*-box is expressed during development. The molecular study of tumour cells which show cytogenetic evidence of amplified DNA, but where amplification of known proto-oncogene has not been detected, could represent a novel strategy for identifying as-yet unknown genes involved in growth control and able to contribute to carcinogenesis.

Great potential for understanding both neuroblastoma development and neural differentiation lies in defining the genetic information apparently deleted on chromosome 1. Deletions of genetic material have been found by cytogenetic analysis in several types of tumours (for review see [48]) and they are thought to indicate loss of cellular genes involved in the control of specific differentiation pathways. Genetic information of this kind has been termed 'tumour suppressor' genes. At this point there should be no doubt that a deeper understanding of the function of oncogenes and tumour suppressor genes could lead to further understanding of tumorigenesis.

ACKNOWLEDGEMENT

I am grateful to I. Ulbrich for rapid and skilful typing of the manuscript.

REFERENCES

[1] Brodeur, G. M., Sekhon, G. S. & Goldstein, M. N. (1975). Specific chromosomal aberrations in human neuroblastoma. *Am. J. Hum. Genet.* **27** 20A
[2] Hansen, M. F. & Cavanee, W. K. (1987). Genetics of cancer predisposition. *Cancer Res.* **47** 5518–5527
[3] Cox, D., Yuncken, C. & Spriggs, A. (1965). Minute chromatin bodies in malignant tumours of childhood. *Lancet* **2** 55–58
[4] Levan, A., Levan, G. & Mitelman, F. (1977). Chromosomes and cancer. *Hereditas* **86** 15–30
[5] Cowell, J. K. (1982). Double minutes and homogeneously staining chromosomal regions: gene amplification in mammalian cells. *Annu. Rev. Genet.* **16** 21–59
[6] Barker, P. E. (1982). Double minutes in human tumor cells. *Cancer Genet. Cytogenet.* **5** 81–94
[7] Biedler, J. L., Helson, L. & Spengler, B. S. (1973) *Cancer Res.* **33** 2543–2652
[8] Schimke, R. T. (1984). Gene amplification in cultured animal cells. *Cell* **37** 705–713
[9] Kanda, N., Schreck, R., Alt, F., Bruns, G., Baltimore, D. & Latt, S. (1983). Isolation of amplified DNA sequences from IMR-32 human neuroblastoma cells: facilitation by fluorescence-activated flow sorting of metaphase chromosome. *Proc. Natl. Acad. Sci. USA* **80** 4069–4073

[10] Brodeur, G. M., Green, A. A. & Hayes, F. A. (1981). Cytogenetic features of human neuroblastomas and cell lines. *Cancer Res.* **41** 4678–4686
[11] Alitalo, K. & Schwab, M. (1986). Oncogene amplification in tumour cells. *Adv. Cancer Res.* **47** 235–279
[12] Schwab, M. (1985). Amplification of N-myc in human neuroblastomas. *Trends Genet.* **1** 271–275
[13] Schwab, M., Alitalo, K., Klempnauer, K. H., Varmus, H. E., Bishop, J. M., Gilbert, F., Brodeur, G., Goldstein, M. & Trent, J. (1983). Amplified DNA with limited homology to *myc* cellular oncogene is shared by human neuroblastoma cell lines and a neuroblastoma tumor. *Nature* **305** 245–248
[14] Kohl, N. E., Kanda, N., Schreck, R. R., Bruns, G., Latt, S. A., Gilbert, F. & Alt, F. (1983). Transposition and amplification of oncogene-related sequence in human neuroblastomas. *Cell* **35** 359–367
[15] Shiloh, Y., Rose, E., Colletti-Feener, C., Korf, B., Kaukel, L. M. & Latt, S. A. (1987). Rapid cloning of multiple amplified neucleotide sequences from human neuroblastoma cell lines by phenol emulsion competitive DNA reassociation. *Gene* **51** 53–59
[16] Shiloh, Y., Shipley, J., Brodeur, G., Bruns, G., Korf, B., Donlon, T., Schreck, R. R., Seeger, T., Sakai, K. & Latt, S. A. (1985). Differential amplification, assembly, and relocation of multiple DNA sequences in human neuroblastomas and neuroblastoma cell lines. *Proc. Natl. Acad. Sci. USA* **82** 3761–3765
[17] Shiloh, Y., Korf, B., Kohl, N. E., Sakai, K., Brodeur, G. M., Harris, P., Kanda, N., Seeger, R. C., Alt, F. W. & Latt, S. A. (1986). Amplification and rearrangement of DNA sequences from the chromosomal region 2p24 in human neuroblastomas. *Cancer Res.* **46** 5297–5301
[18] Schwab, M. (1988). Myc-box genes: N-myc and L-myc. In: T. Curran, S. Prenreddy & A. Skalka (eds.) *Oncogene Handbook*, in press
[19] Nau, M. M., Brooks, B. J., Battey, J., Gazdar, A., Kirsch, I., McBride, O. W., Bertnes, V., Hollis, G. F. & Minna, J. D. (1985). L-myc, a new myc-related gene amplified and expressed in human small cell lung cancer. *Nature* **318** 69–73
[20] Brooks, B., Battey, J., Nau, M. M., Gazdar, A. & Minna, J. (1987). Amplification and expression of the myc gene in small cell lung cancer. In: G. Klein (ed.) *Advances in Viral Oncology* vol. 7, Raven Press, New York, pp. 155–172
[21] Dalla-Favera, R., Bregni, M., Erikson, J., Patterson, D., Gallo, R. C. & Croce, C. (1982). Human c-myc oncogene is located on the region of chromosome 8 that is translocated in Burkitt lymphoma cells. *Proc. Natl. Acad. Sci. USA* **79** 7824–7827
[22] Schwab, M., Varmus, H. E., Bishop, J. M., Grzeschik, K. H., Naylor, S., Sakaguchi, A., Brodeur, G. & Trent, J. (1984). Chromosome localization in normal human cells and neuroblastomas of a gene releated to c-myc. *Nature* **308** 288–291
[23] Nau, M. M., Brooks, B., Carney, D., Gazdar, A., Battey, J., Sausville, E. & Minna, J. (1986). Human small cell lung cancers show amplification and expression of the N-myc gene. *Proc. Natl. Acad. Sci. USA* **83** 1092–1096
[24] Lee, W. H., Murphee, A. C. & Benedict, W. F. (1984). Expression and amplification of the N-myc gene in primary retinoblastoma. *Nature* **309** 458–460
[25] Squire, J., Gallie, B. L. & Phillips, R. A. (1985). A detailed analysis of

chromosomal changes in heritable and non-heritable retinoblastoma. *Hum. Genet.* **70** 291–301

[26] Garson, J. A., McIntyre, P. G. & Kemshead, J. T. (1985). N-myc amplification in malignant astrocytoma. *Lancet* (September 28) 718–719

[27] Stanton, L. W., Schwab, M. & Bishop, J. M. (1986). Nucleotide sequence of the human N-myc. *Proc. Natl. Acad. Sci. USA* **83** 1771–1776

[28] Kohl, N. E., Legouy, E., De Pincho, R. A., Nisen, P. D., Smith, R. K., Gee, C. E. & Alt, F. W. (1986). Human N-myc is closely related in organization and nucleotide sequence to c-myc. *Nature* **319** 73–77

[29] Slamon, D. J., Boone, T. C., Seeger, R. C., Keith, D. E., Chaziu, V., Lee, H. C. & Souza, L. M. (1986). Identification and characterization of the protein encoded by the human N-myc oncogene. *Science* **232** 768–772

[30] Ramsay, G., Stanton, L., Schwab, M. & Bishop, J. M. (1986). N-myc encodes a nuclear protein that binds to DNA. *Molec. Cell Biol.* **6** 4450–4457

[31] Schwab, M., Varmus, H. E. & Bishop, J. M. (1985). The human N-myc gene contributes to tumorigenic conversion of mammalian cells in culture. *Nature* **316** 160–162

[32] Schwab, M. & Bishop, J. M. (in press). High ectopic expression of N-myc establishes primary rat embryo cells in culture. *Proc. Natl. Acad. Sci. USA*.

[33] Small, M., Hay, N., Ramsay, G., Schwab, M. & Bishop, J. M. (1987). N-myc induces tumorigenic conversion of cultured rat cells. *Molec. Cell Biol.* **7** 1638–1645

[34] Jakobovits, A., Schwab, M., Bishop, J. M. & Martin, G. (1985). Expression of N-myc in teratocarcinoma stem cells and mouse embryos. *Nature* **318**, 188–191

[35] Schwab, M., Ellison, J., Busch, M., Rosenau, W., Varmus, H. E. & Bishop, J. M. (1984). Enhanced expression of the human gene N-myc consequent to amplification of DNA may contribute to malignant progression of neuroblastoma. *Proc. Natl. Acad. Sci. USA* **81** 4940–4944

[36] Zimmerman, K. A., Yancopoulos, G. D., Collum, R. G., Smith, R. K., Kohl, N. E., Denis, K. A., Nau, M. M., Witte, O., Toran-Allerand, D., Gee, C. E., Minna, J. D. & Alt, F. (1986). Differential expression of myc-family genes during murine development. *Nature* **319** 780–783

[37] Squire, J., Goddard, A. D., Canton, M., Becher, A., Phillips, R. A. & Gallie, B. L. (1986). Tumours induction by the retinoblastoma mutation is independent of N-myc expression. *Nature* **327** 555–557

[38] Nisen, R. D., Zimmerman, K. A., Cotter, S. V., Gilbert, F. & Alt, F. W. (1986). Enhanced expression of the N-myc gene in Wilm's tumors. *Cancer Res.* **46** 6217–6222

[39] Grady, E. F., Schwab, M. & Rosenau, W. (1987). Expression of N-myc and c-src during the development of fetal human brain. *Cancer Res.* **47** 2931–2936

[40] Muller, R., Tremblay, J. M., Adamson, E. D. & Verma, I. M. (1983). Tissue and cell-type specific expression of two human c-onc genes. *Nature* **304** 454–456

[41] Thiele, C. J., Reynolds, C. P. & Israel, M. (1985). Decreased expression of N-myc precedes retinoic acid-induced morphological differentiation of human neuroblastoma. *Nature* **313** 404–406

[42] Brodeur, J., Seeger, R. C., Schwab, M., Varmus, H. E. & Bishop, J. M.

(1984). Amplification of N-myc in untreated human neuroblastoma correlates with advanced disease stage, *Science,* **224** 1121–1124

[43] Seeger, R. C., Brodeur, G. M., Sather, H., Dalton, A., Siegel, S. E., Wong, K. Y. & Hammond, D. (1985). Association of multiple copies of the N-myc oncogene with rapid progression of neuroblastomas. *N. Engl. J. Med.* **313** 1111–1116

[44] Foulds, L. (1958). The natural history of cancer. *J. Chronic Dis.* **8** 2–37

[45] Nowell, P. (1976). The clonal evolution of tumor cell populations. *Science* **194** 23–28

[46] Sager, R., Gadi, I. K., Stephens, L. & Grabwy, C. T., (1985). Gene amplification: an example of accelerated evolution in tumorigenic cells. *Proc. Natl. Acad. Sci. USA* **82** 7015–7019

[47] Becker, L. E. & Hinton, D. (1983). Primitive neuroectodermal tumors of the central nervous system. *Hum. Path.* **14** 538–550

[48] Yunis, J. (1986). *Important Adv. Oncol.* **2** 93–128

4

Phenotypes of neuroblastoma cells as distinguished by monoclonal antibodies

Takafumi Matsumura[*†], Tohru Sugimoto[‡] and Tadashi Sawada[*]
Department of Pediatrics* and Children's Research Hospital[‡], Kyoto Prefectural University of Medicine, Kamikyoku, Kyoto 602, Japan; and Pediatric Division[†], Red Cross Hospital, Maizuri, Kyoto 624, Japan

1. INTRODUCTION

Neuroblastoma can be confused clinically and histologically with other 'small round cell' tumours, namely Wilm's tumour, rhabdomyosarcoma, lymphoma and, especially, Ewing's sarcoma and primitive neuroectodermal tumours [1–3]. In particular, when the metastatic site is the first observable focus of the tumour's existence, the differential diagnosis of one small round cell tumour from another is very difficult to make. On the basis of the present clinical, histological, and biochemical features of neuroblastoma [4], more than a few cases remain unclassified or are misdiagnosed.

Recent developments in immunohistochemical and immunocytochemical techniques have provided new tools for the differential diagnosis of neuroblastoma from the other small round cell tumours. The identities of many of the monoclonal antibodies bound to neuroblastoma cells have been established [5–7] and, through the use of various monoclonal antibodies, neuroblastoma cells have been well characterized and can be distinguished from other tumour cells [8–13]. Most of the antibodies, however, are not exclusively specific for neuroblastoma, but cross-react with other tumours and tissues as well. In this regard, immunocytochemically, by using a single monoclonal antibody, it is impossible to distinguish neuroblastoma cells from other tumour cells. A panel of several monoclonal antibodies highly specific for neuroblastoma cells is required for the accurate diagnosis of neuroblastoma.

In this chapter, we will review monoclonal antibodies bound to neuroblastoma cells and identify the immunological membrane phenotype of neuroblastoma cells by using a panel of monoclonal antibodies. Immunocytochemical studies, augmenting histological and biochemical studies, can contribute to accurate and rapid diagnosis of neuroblastoma for selection of appropriate therapy. Further information may make it possible to subclassify neuroblastomas into groups of differentiation stages and to evaluate prognosis of the disease.

2. MONOCLONAL ANTIBODIES BOUND TO NEUROBLASTOMA CELLS

The most important consideration, when using a monoclonal antibody, is its specificity to certain tumour cells. More than 50 monoclonal antibodies have been reported to bind to neuroblastoma cells since the first monoclonal antibody PI153/3 was described by Kennett and Gilbert in 1979 [14]. Unfortunately, however, no truly neuroblastoma-specific monoclonal antibody has yet been reported. About half of the identified monoclonal antibodies were raised by immunization with neuroblastoma cells; however, another half of them were raised against other neuroectodermally derived tumours and tissues, haemotopoietic cells, lung cancer cells, and so forth. They reveal non-specific cross-reactions not only with tumour cells but with normal cells and tissues as well. The major characteristics of monoclonal antibodies bound to neuroblastoma cells are listed in Tables 1–4 according to the source of immunogen. As well as these antibodies, there are also those raised against lung cancer cell lines [6,59,60].

As listed in Table 1, more than 20 monoclonal antibodies were raised against neuroblastoma cell lines. All of these antibodies were highly reactive to cell lines and fresh samples of neuroblastoma. Most of them, however, have been also reported to bind to other small round cell tumours, namely, rhabdomyosarcoma, Ewing's sarcoma, Wilms' tumour, leukaemia and lymphoma. The antibody 5A7 only did not bind to any of the tumour samples examined; however, it did cross-react with primitive neuroectodermal tumour and some normal tissues (colon and kidney in adult; adrenal medulla in foetus) [25]. This suggests that no truly neuroblastoma-specific antigen has been found so far by means of monoclonal antibodies.

For the present, a panel of monoclonal antibodies highly specific to neuroblastoma cells should be used for the accurate diagnosis of neuroblastoma. Recently, a world-wide cooperative study for the screening of monoclonal antibodies bound to neuroblastoma cells was organized by Dr. J. T. Kemshead, Imperial Cancer Research Fund Laboratory, London. At the meeting on Advances in Neuroblastoma Research in Philadelphia, 1987, Dr. Kemshead reported tentatively that four antibodies, UJ13A, 3F8, 126.4, and 5.1.H11, were the most highly reactive to neuroblastoma cells among over 50 monoclonal antibodies registered [61]. However, since these four antibodies also had cross-reactivities with other tumour cells, further analysis is necessary to isolate the specific antibodies.

Such cross-reactivities are, however, neither unusual nor surprising. Cell membrane structures are similar among various human cells, neoplastic or normal, and furthermore some alterations in membrane structure are considered to occur in association with malignant progression. Another aspect seems to indicate that such cross-reaction demonstrates an oncodevelopmental relationship. Many monoclonal antibodies bound to neuroblastoma cells also cross-react with other neuroectodermally derived tumours and tissues, since they have been raised by immunization with these tumours and tissues. These observations indicate that neuroectodermally

Table 1 — Monoclonal antibodies raised against neuroblastoma

Monoclonal antibody	Immunogen (cell line)	Antigen identified	Reactivity with[a]					Reference
			NB	RMS	EW	WT	LL	
PI153/3	IMR6	gp20K	+(49/55)				+(16/47)	[14]
C10.115	LA-N-1	ND	+(14/16)	−(0/1)			+(6/13)	[15]
M1/N1	CHP100		+(6/12)				+(2/7)	[16]
HSAN1.2	SMS-SAN	ND	+(30/30)	−(0/2)	+(1/2)	+(2/2)	−(0/44)	[17]
3F8	Not clarified	ggGD2	+(27/29)	+(3/6)	+(1/6)	+(2/6)	+(1/31)	[18]
2F7	Not clarified	ggGD2	+(6/8)	+(2/6)	−(0/6)	−(0/6)	+(1/31)	[18]
3A7	Not clarified	ggGD2	+(27/29)	+(2/6)	−(0/6)	−(0/6)	+(1/31)	[18]
3G6	Not clarified	ggGD2	+(27/29)	+(3/6)	−(0/6)	+(1/6)	+(1/31)	[18]
6-19	Mixed cells	ND	+(12/12)	+(1/1)	+(1/1)	+(1/1)	−(0/9)	[19,20]
6-3	(SK-N-MC etc.)	ND	+(12/12)					[19]
5-5	(SK-N-MC)	ND	+(6/6)					[19]
MC25	SK-N-MC	ND	+(15/17)	−(0/3)	+(1/1)		−(0/16)	[21]
MC139	SK-N-MC	gp35K	+(10/10)	+(2/2)	+(1/1)		+(8/18)	[22]
CE7	IMR-32	gp190K	+(22/22)				−(0/4)	[23]
CB10	IMR-32	gp180K	+(11/22)				−(0/4)	[23]
AD2	IMR-32	ND	+(15/22)				−(0/4)	[23]
BC1	IMR-32	ND	+(8/9)				+(2/3)	[23]
BC4	IMR-32	ND	+(5/9)				−(0/3)	[23]
5G3	SK-N-AS	gp200,215K	+(6/7)	−(0/1)	−(0/1)		−(0/6)	[24]
5A7	LA-N-1	gp65-67K	+(30/31)	−(0/4)	−(0/8)	−(0/2)	−(0/21)	[25]
14.18	LA-N-1	ggGD2	+(8/8)		+(1/1)		−(0/4)	[26]
KP-NAC2	KP-N-RT	gp66-68K	+(42/43)	+(1/4)	−(0/3)	−(0/6)	+(3/65)	[27]
KP-NAC8	KP-N-RT	gp200K	+(41/43)	−(0/4)	+(1/3)	−(0/6)	+(2/65)	[27,28]
KP-NAC9	KP-N-RT	ND	+(42/43)	+(2/4)	+(2/3)	+(3/6)	+(2/65)	[27]
KP-NAC10	KP-N-RT	ND	+(41/43)	−(0/4)	−(0/3)	+(1/6)	+(39/65)	[27]

gp, glycoprotein; gg, ganglioside; ND, not determined; NB, neuroblastoma; RMS, rhabdomyosarcoma; EW, Ewing's sarcoma, WT, Wilms' tumour, LL, lymphoma–leukaemia.

[a] Numbers in parentheses are the numbers of positive and of total cell lines in the clinical samples originally reported.

Table 2 — Monoclonal antibodies bound to neuroblastoma raised against neuroectodermally derived tumours excluding neuroblastoma

Monoclonal antibody	Immunogen	Antigen identified	Reactivity[a]	Reference
CG-12	Glioblastoma	ND	NB (2/3), GB (17/37), ME (8/9), RMS (0/1), LL (0/4)	[29,30]
G13-C6	Glioblastoma	ND	NB (1/3). GB (9/13), ME (5/5)	[29,31]
81C6	Glioma	pp210,230K	NB (1/3), GB (24/27), ME (5/11), RMS (1/1), WT (1/1), LL (0/6)	[32]
2F3	Glioma	ND	NB (2/3), GB (5/12), RMS (0/1), WT (0/1), LL (3/4)	[33]
4C7	Glioma	ND	NB (2/3), GB (4/12), RMS (0/1), WT (0/1), LL (1/4)	[33]
5B7	Glioma	ND	NB (2/3), GB (4/12), RMS (0/1), WT (0/1), LL (2/4)	[33]
AJ225	Astrocytoma	145K	NB (1/2), ME (1/10), LL (1/3)	[34]
AO10	Astrocytoma	gp110K	NB (2/2), ME (3/10), LL (1/2)	[34]
AJ9	Astrocytoma	ND	NB (2/2), ME (10/10), LL (0/3)	[34]
AJ17	Astrocytoma	ND	NB (1/2), ME (10/10), LL (0/3)	[34]
AJ425	Astrocytoma	ND	NB (2/2), ME (10/10), LL (3/3)	[34]
K117	Astrocytoma	gp25K	NB (10/10), ME (2/2), EW (2/2), RMS (2/2), LL (1/18)	[22]
7.51	Melanoma	ND	NB (+), ME (+), GB (+)	[35]
7.60	Melanoma	ND	NB (+), ME (+), GB (+)	[35]
376	Melanoma	ND	NB (10/10), ME (4/4), RMS (1/1)	[36]
Mel-5	Melanoma	ND	NB (3/3), ME (11/11), LL (0/12), GB (+)	[30]
Mel-14	Melonoma	ND	NB (1/3), ME (11/11), LL (0/12), GB (+)	[30]
Me3-TB7	Melanoma	ND	NB (3/3), ME (10/11), LL (0/12), GB (+)	[30]
Me4-F8	Melanoma	ND	NB (3/3), ME (10/11), LL (0/8), GB(+)	[30]
Me5-D5	Melanoma	ND	NB (3/3), ME (10/11), LL (0/8), GB(+)	[30]
705F6	Melanoma	95K	NB (+), ME (+), LL (3/7)	[37]
L55	Melanoma	gg	NB (7/8); ME (18/36), LL (1/14), G (6/8)	[38]
L72	Melanoma	ggGD2	NB (5/8), ME (21/36), LL (0/14), G (6/8)	[38,39]
ME20.4	Melanoma	gp75K	NB (+), ME (+)	[40]
DW-1	PNET	ND	NB (10/21), PNET (1/6), RMS (0/1), LL (0/5), ME (3/5)	[41]

gp, glycoprotein; gg, ganglioside; ND, not determined; NB, neuroblastoma; RMS, rhabdomyosarcoma; EW, Ewing's sarcoma; WT, Wilm's tumour; LL, lymphoma–leukaemia; GB, glioblastoma; ME, melanoma; G, glioma; PNET, primitive neuroectodermal tumour.

[a] Numbers in parenthesis are the numbers of positive and of total cell lines in the clinical samples originally reported.

Table 3 — Monoclonal antibodies bound to neuroblastoma raised against neuroectodermally derived tissues

Monoclonal antibody	Immunogen	Antigen identified	Reactivity[a]	Reference
A2B5	Chicken retina	ggGQ	NB (23/30), LL (3/11)	[42]
anti-Thy-1	Purified Thy-1	25K,Thy-1	NB (4/4), LL (0/2), EW (0/2), WT (0/2)	[43]
390	Foetal brain	25K,Thy-1	NB (9/10), ME (1/4), RMS (1/1), GB (2/3)	[44]
UJ127:11	Foetal brain	220-240K	NB(+)	[45]
UJ13A	Foetal brain	ND	NB (66/76), LL (3/129), WT (3/3), EW (0/3), RMS (2/3)	[46]
UJ308	Foetal brain	180–200K	NB (+), LL (+)	[47]
7H10c14	Foetal brain	ND	NB (1/1), GB (+), LL (+)	[48,49]
4D2c16	Foetal brain	ND	NB (1/1), GB (+), LL (−)	[49]
1H8c12	Foetal brain	ND	NB (2/3), GB (9/14), ME (0/2), RMS (0/1), LL (0/4)	[48]
1H8c13	Foetal brain	ND	NB (2/3), GB (7/14), ME (1/2), RMS (0/1), LL (0/4)	[48]
44	Foetal brain	ND	NB (+), LL (+)	[6]
11-1	Isolated antigen of PI153/3		NB (+), LL (+)	[6]
25-6	Isolated antigen of PI153/3		NB (+), LL (+)	[6]

gp, glycoprotein; gg, ganglioside; ND, not determined; NB, neuroblastoma; RMS, rhabdomyosarcoma; EW, Ewing's sarcoma; WT, Wilm's tumour; LL, lymphoma–leukaemia; GB, glioblastoma; ME, melanoma; G, glioma; PNET, primitive neuroectodermal tumour.

[a] Numbers in parenthesis are the numbers of positive and of total cell lines in the clinical samples originally reported.

Table 4 — Monoclonal antibodies bound to neuroblastoma raised against haematopoietic cells

Monoclonal antibody	Immunogen	Antigen identified	Reactivity[a]	Reference
NA1-34	Thymocyte	45-49K+12K	NB (+), LL (+), ME (−)	[47,50]
OKT-6	Thymocyte	45-49K+12K	NB (2/2), LL (+)	[47,51]
OKT 9	Thymocyte	180K	NB (2/2), LL (+), ME (+)	[47,51]
BA-1	pre-B-ALL	ND	NB (+), LL (+), ME (+)	[52]
BA-2	pre-B-ALL	24K	NB (+), LL (+), ME (+)	[53]
HNK-1(Leu-7)	T-cell	110K	NB (26/32), EW (6/10), ME (2/2), LL (+)	[54]
ALB7	ALL	ND	NB (+), LL (+)	[55]
ALB8	ALL	ND	NB (+), LL (+)	[55]
ALB9	ALL	ND	NB (+), LL (+)	[55]
SJ-9A4	ALL	24K	NB (8/8), EW (9/1), LL (7/18)	[56]
L368	B-cell	β2m	NB (2/4), LL (+)	[57]
W6/32	Lymphocyte	HLA-A,B,C	NB (2/4), LL (+)	[57]
FMG25	T-lymphoma	ND	NB (45/47), EW (0/14), LL (5/54), RMS (0/15)	[58]

gp, glycoprotein; gg, ganglioside; ND, not determined; NB, neuroblastoma; RMS, rhabdomyosarcoma; EW, Ewing's sarcoma; WT, Wilm's tumour; LL, lymphoma–leukaemia; GB, glioblastoma; ME, melanoma; G, glioma; PNET, primitive neuroectodermal tumour.

[a] Numbers in parenthesis are the numbers of positive and of total cell lines in the clinical samples originally reported.

derived cells have either the same molecules or the same antigenic determinants expressed on the cell surface membrane. Therefore, when considering the usefulness of a monoclonal antibody, it is necessary to characterize the biochemical and biological significance of the antigen recognized by a monoclonal antibody. Unfortunately, in many cases these characterizations remain undefined.

Actually, it has become easy to produce various monoclonal antibodies by using recently developed techniques; however, greater efforts should be made to determine the biochemical and biological significance of each antigen defined by the monoclonal antibody.

3. HETEROGENEITY IN MEMBRANE PHENOTYPES OF NEUROBLASTOMA CELLS

In a broad classification of the monoclonal antibodies bound to neuroblastoma cells, none of them reacts with either all of the neuroblastoma cell lines or all of the clinical samples. Several studies of the membrane phenotypes of neuroblastoma cells, using a panel of monoclonal antibodies, have demonstrated considerable heterogeneity in antigen expression among cell lines and fresh samples. Antigenic heterogeneity, which was initially observed in neuroblastoma cell lines with the M1/N1 antibody [16], has also been demonstrated in fresh neuroblastoma samples [16,62]. These results indicate either a qualitative or a quantitative heterogeneity in antigenic expression. With regard to heterogeneity, particularly in quantity, the binding assay system used should be specified, because different assay systems have different sensitivities for detection of antigens.

In our laboratory, we characterized membrane phenotypes of various neuroblastoma cell lines by using a large panel of monoclonal antibodies with indirect immunofluorescence. The results are summarized in Fig. 1. Seven of twenty human neuroblastoma cell lines (KP-N-RTLN, KP-N-SIFA, KP-N-SILA2B4, KP-N-RTBM, KP-N-YN, SK-N-SH, and NB-1) exhibited a similar reactivity pattern, while thirteen cell lines had various reactivity patterns, indicating the heterogeneity in membrane phenotypes of neuroblastoma cells. Among these cell lines, the KP-N-RTBMV line is a variant derived from the KP-N-RTBM parent line after long-term cultures. The KP-N-RTBMV line revealed a different membrane phenotype and a different biological nature from the parent line, which included anchorage-dependent and anchorage-independent growth, transplantability to the nude mouse, and reactivity to differentiation agents (unpublished data). A similar phenomenon has been observed *in vivo*. The KCN or KCNR line, which was established before or after therapy by Reynolds *et al.* [63], also revealed a heterogeneity in membrane phenotype. These observations suggest that either long-term culture or anticancer agents may induce alterations of cell surface membrane antigens, and that these heterogeneities in membrane phenotype may correlate with reactivity to anticancer agents. In another example, KP-N-SILA2B4 (LA2B4) and KP-N-SILA2D2 (LA2D2) were sublines with distinctive morphological phenotypes, derived from the KP-N-SILA parent line which was established from the same metastasis of a patient with neuroblastoma in our laboratory. Morphologically, the LA2B4 line is a neuronal (neuroblastic (N)) type, and the LA2D2 line is an epithelial (substrate-adherent(S)) type. These two lines also have distinctive membrane phenotypes in

Monoclonal antibody \ Neuroblastoma cell line	KP-N-RTLN	KP-N-SIFA	KP-N-SILA2B4	KP-N-RTBM	KP-N-YN	SK-N-SH	NB-1	SK-N-AS	KP-N-AY	SMS-KCNR	SK-N-DZ	SMS-KAN	SMS-KCN	GOTO	SJ-N-KP	SK-N-FI	KP-N-RTBMV	SJ-N-CG	SK-N-LO	KP-N-SILA2D2
A2B5	●	●	●	●	●	●	●	●	●	●	●	●	●	●	●	●	●	●	●	●
BA-2	●	●	●	●	●	●	●	●	●	●	●	●	●	●	●	●	●	●	●	◎
anti-Thy-1	●	●	●	●	●	●	●	●	●	●	●	●	●	●	●	●	●	◎	●	●
UJ13A	●	●	●	●	●	●	●	●	●	●	●	●	●	●	●	●	●	●	○	●
KP-NAC9	●	●	●	●	●	●	●	●	●	●	●	●	●	●	●	●	●	○	●	●
UJ127:11	●	●	●	●	●	●	●	●	●	●	●	●	●	●	●	●	○	●	●	●
BA-1.	●	●	●	●	●	●	●	●	●	●	●	●	●	●	●	●	●	●	○	○
PI153/3	●	●	●	●	●	●	●	●	●	●	●	●	●	●	●	●	●	●	○	○
KP-NAC10	●	●	●	●	●	●	●	●	●	●	●	●	●	●	●	○	●	●	○	○
HSAN1.2	●	●	●	●	●	●	●	●	●	●	●	●	●	●	●	○	●	○	●	○
Leu7	●	●	●	●	●	●	●	●	●	●	●	●	●	●	○	●	○	●	●	○
KP-NAC2	●	●	●	●	●	●	◎	●	●	●	●	●	●	○	●	●	○	●	●	○
KP-NAC8	●	●	●	●	●	◎	◎	●	●	●	◎	◎	◎	●	●	●	●	○	○	●
BBM1	●	●	●	●	●	●	●	●	●	◎	○	○	○	●	●	●	●	●	●	●
W6/32	●	●	●	◎	◎	●	●	●	○	○	○	○	○	●	●	●	●	●	●	●
ME20.4	●	●	●	●	●	●	●	○	○	○	●	○	○	●	●	●	●	●	●	◎
J5	○	○	○	○	○	○	○	○	○	○	○	○	○	○	○	○	○	●	○	○
OKIa-1	○	○	○	○	○	○	○	○	○	○	○	○	○	○	○	○	○	○	○	○
GAP8.3	○	○	○	○	○	○	○	○	○	○	○	○	○	○	○	○	○	○	○	○
Genox3.53	○	○	○	○	○	○	○	○	○	○	○	○	○	○	○	○	○	○	○	○

● Positive cells $\geqq$ 25% ◎ Positive cells $\geqq$ 10% ○ Positive cells < 10%

Fig. 1 — Cell surface membrane phenotypes of human neuroblastoma cell lines determined by indirect immunofluorescence. At least 200 cells were examined under an ultraviolet microscope, and the percentage of stained cells showing either negative or positive ring staining was counted. The results were determined by the mean value of three to five independent experiments.

antigen expression associated with morphological distinctions (Fig. 2). Similar observations have been described in other neuroblastoma cell lines [64,65]. Immunocytochemically, Rettig *et al.* [65] have confirmed the neuronal phenotype of N-type cells and demonstrated that S-type cells had a non-neuronal phenotype closely resembling the phenotype of cultured ectomesenchymal cells. These two types of cells undergo morphological interconversion, termed transdifferentiation, sponta-

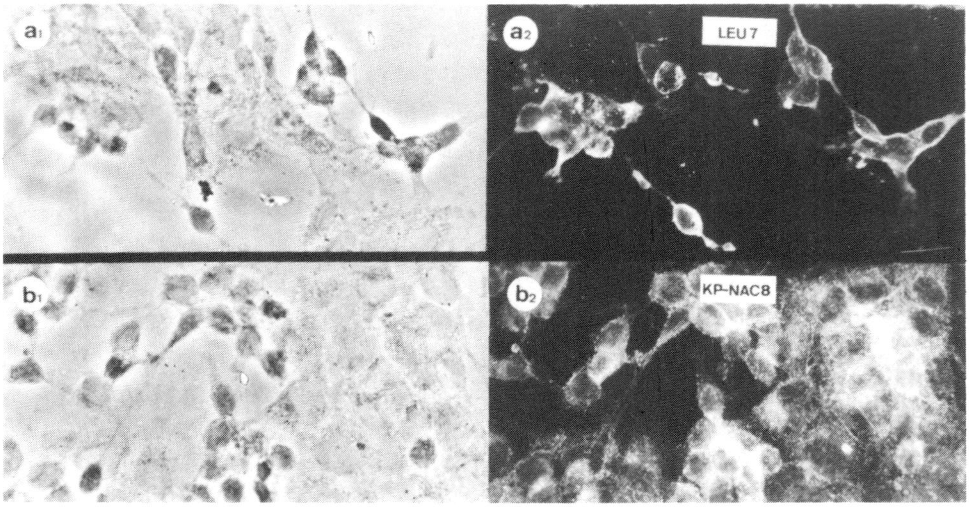

Fig. 2 — Photomicrographs of KP-N-SILA cells. a_1,b_1, phase-contrast microscopy; a_2b_2, indirect immunofluorescence with Leu7 (a_2) and KP-NAC8 (b_2). Morphologically epithelial-type cells were reactive to Leu7; in contrast, neuronal-type cells were not (a_1,a_2). Both types of cells were reactive to KP-NAC8 (b_1,b_2).

neously in culture. In our observations, the LA2B4 cells of N type transdifferentiated to S-type cells, and the LA2D2 cells of S type have a phenotype closely resembling that of Schwann cells examined in ganglioneuroma tissues (data not shown). Accordingly, these observations may suggest a possible relationship between immunological membrane phenotypes and morphological phenotypes of neuroblastoma cells, particularly in association with differentiation. Actually, however, no definitive correlation between membrane phenotypes and the biological nature of neuroblastoma cells has been proven.

Many researchers have investigated alterations of membrane phenotypes associated with chemically induced differentiation *in vitro*, in order to define differentiation antigens of neuroblastoma cells [66–68]. Nevertheless, for the present, the existence of differentiation antigens, has not been demonstrated in neuroblastoma cells. If differentiation antigens can be identified, they could prove useful in the choice of appropriate therapy and in the prediction of prognosis of the disease.

Finally, no universal membrane phenotype has been found among neuroblastoma cells, and eventually membrane phenotypes might even be found to have differences as individual as human faces. Fortunately, however, a certain tendency is evident as described in Fig. 1. Three antibodies, A2B5, BA-2 and anti-Thy-1, each reacted with all 20 neuroblastoma cell lines. Antibodies UJ13A, KP-NAC9, UJ127:11, BA-1, PI153/3, KP-NAC10, HSAN1.2, Leu7, KP-NAC2, KP-NAC8, BBM1, W6/32 and ME20.4 bound to all except between one to five of the neuroblastoma cell lines. Accordingly, by using 16 of these monoclonal antibodies, it is possible to identify tumour cells as neuroblastoma cells with a high probability. In particular, among these antibodies, 13 monoclonal antibodies not including BBM1,

W6/32 and ME20.4 were reactive to the 13 morphologically neuronal-type cell lines, while they were variably reactive to epithelial-type cell lines. Our examination with clinical samples also demonstrated that this panel of 13 monoclonal antibodies reacted with all 26 fresh neuroblastoma samples taken from tumour tissue or bone marrow metastases. Consequently, neuroblastoma cells may be defined to have the standard membrane phenotype that was expressed by their binding to these 13 antibodies, although it seems likely that the phenotype may alter according to morphological variation, long-term cultures or chemical agents.

4. DISCRIMINATION OF NEUROBLASTOMA FROM OTHER SMALL ROUND CELL TUMOURS

Using the same panel of monoclonal antibodies, we compared the membrane phenotype of neuroblastoma cells with those of other small round cell tumours, namely rhabdomyosarcoma, Wilms' tumour and Ewing's sarcoma, for differential diagnosis. As summarized in Fig. 3, a greater variation in heterogeneity was observed in these tumour cell lines than in the neuroblastoma cell lines. A2B5, BA-2, and anti-Thy-1 bound to all neuroblastoma lines examined, but they also all cross-reacted variably with the rhabdomyosarcoma, Wilm's tumour and Ewing's sarcoma lines examined. Using only three of these antibodies, it is impossible to discriminate between neuroblastoma and these small round cell tumours. In contrast, as BA-1, PI153/3 and KP-NAC10 did not bind to the tumour lines examined, they can be useful for distinguishing these tumour cells from neuroblastoma cells. They all, however, cross-reacted with haematopoietic cells, as described in Table 1. One should pay attention to discrimination between neuroblastoma and haemotopoietic malignancies. Leu-7, KP-NAC2, and KP-NAC8 should prove useful to distinguish Wilm's tumour from neuroblastoma, because they did not bind to any of the four Wilm's tumour lines tested.

Even though the present data are the results from a limited sampling, they demonstrate that there are as many cell lines as there are membrane phenotypes. Although all of these antibodies have high reactivity with neuroblastoma, in various degrees they lack true specificity to neuroblastoma. It is evident that there are also as many monoclonal antibodies as there are cross-reactivities. At the present time, we must make free use of the abundant antibodies, and choose the most useful panel of antibodies of differential diagnosis with the minimum number of antibodies. The present results suggest that positive bindings to antibodies A2B5, BA-2, and anti-Thy-1 are also necessary for affirmation of neuroblastoma, and that positive bindings to antibodies BA-1, PI153/3, and KP-NAC10 are necessary for confirmation that the tumour cells are not rhabdomyosarcoma, Wilm's tumour or Ewing's sarcoma. Furthermore, reactivities with other antibodies should support the obtained differential diagnosis.

5. MEMBRANE PHENOTYPE OF FOETAL NEUROBLASTS AS THE ORIGIN OF NEUROBLASTOMA CELLS

Neuroblastoma is thought to arise from primitive sympathetic neuroblasts in the adrenal gland or the sympathetic ganglion that failed to undergo normal differentia-

Cell line / Monoclonal antibody	Rhabdomyosarcoma				Wilms' tumour				Ewing's sarcoma			
	RD	SMS-CTR	A204	A673	SK-NEP-1	G401	SCMC-W1	Wo	TC71	SK-ES-1	SCMC-ES-1	RD-ES
A2B5	●	○	○	○	NT	○	○	●	●	●	NT	NT
BA-2	●	●	●	○	●	○	○	○	○	○	○	○
anti-Thy-1	●	○	○	●	●	◎	●	●	●	●	●	●
UJ13A	●	●	○	●	●	○	○	○	○	●	○	●
KP-NAC9	●	○	○	●	●	●	●	○	○	●	●	●
UJ127:11	●	○	○	○	●	○	●	○	○	○	●	●
BA-1	○	○	○	○	○	○	○	○	○	○	○	○
PI153/3	○	○	○	○	○	○	○	○	○	○	○	○
KP-NAC10	○	○	○	○	○	○	○	○	○	○	○	○
HSAN1.2	○	○	○	●	●	○	○	●	●	●	○	●
Leu7	○	○	●	●	○	○	○	○	○	●	●	●
KP-NAC2	○	○	○	●	○	○	○	○	●	○	◎	○
KP-NAC8	○	○	○	○	○	○	○	○	◎	○	○	○
BBM1	●	●	●	●	●	NT	●	●	●	●	NT	NT
W6/32	●	●	●	●	●	●	●	●	●	●	●	●
ME20.4	NT	NT	○	●	●	NT	●	●	●	●	NT	NT
J5	◎	◎	○	○	NT	●	○	○	○	○	NT	NT
OKIa-1	○	○	○	○	○	○	○	○	○	○	NT	NT
GAP8.3	○	○	○	○	○	NT	○	○	○	○	NT	NT
Genox3.53	NT	NT	○	○	○	NT	○	○	○	○	NT	NT

● Positive cells $\geqq$ 25% ◎ Positive cells $\geqq$ 10% ○ Positive cells < 10%

NT; not tested

Fig. 3 — Cell surface membrane phenotypes of rhabdomyosarcoma, Wilm's tumour, and Ewing's sarcoma cell lines determined by indirect immunofluorescence.

tion. Although neuroblastoma cells have been thoroughly analysed in immunological studies of cell surface antigens as described above, foetal neuroblasts have not been studied as the precursor of neuroblastoma cells from this point of view. Some distinctions, based on histopathological studies, between neuroblastoma cells and foetal neuroblasts in the adrenal gland have been demonstrated. No differences in cell surface antigen expression, however, have been defined between these two cell types. Immunological distinction between neuroblastoma cells and foetal neuroblasts may contribute to the identification of differentiation antigens on neuroblastoma cells. We examined a membrane phenotype of foetal neuroblasts in the adrenal gland and compared it with a phenotype of neuroblastoma cells using a panel of 18 monoclonal antibodies with indirect immunofluorescence and immunoperoxidase staining. A comparison of the binding of monoclonal antibodies revealed that antibodies KP-NAC2, KP-NAC9, KP-NAC10, PI153/3, HSAN1.2, UJ127:11, UJ13A, A2B5, ME20.4, anti-Thy-1, BA-1, BA-2, and Leu-7 bound to both neuroblastoma cells and foetal neuroblasts. Antibodies J5, OKIa-1, W6/32, and Genox 3.53 did not bind to either of these cells. KP-NAC8 was the only monoclonal antibody that could distinguish foetal neuroblasts from neuroblastoma cells (Figs. 4 and 5). The specificity of KP-NAC8 binding to neuroblastoma cells but not to foetal

Monoclonal antibody	Neuroblastoma cells (n=14)	Foetal neuroblasts (n=5)
	Stage I – IVs	12 – 21th week of gestation
A2B5	●	●
BA-2	●	●
anti-Thy-1	●	●
UJ13A	●	●
KP-NAC9	●	●
UJ127:11	●	●
BA-1	●	●
PI153/3	●	●
KP-NAC10	●	●
HSAN1.2	●	●
Leu7	●	●
KP-NAC2	●	●
KP-NAC8	●	○
W6/32	○	○
ME20.4	●	●
J5	○	○
OKIa-1	○	○
Genox3.53	○	○

● : Positive ○ : Negative

Fig. 4 — Cell surface membrane phenotypes of neuroblastoma cells in fresh tumour tissues, and foetal neuroblasts in the adrenal gland. Non-fixed frozen sections were stained by indirect immunofluorescence and/or the immunoperoxidase technique. If more than 10% of all examined cells were stained, the reactivity of the sample was determined as positive. In all positive samples, more than half of all cells were stained.

neuroblasts should yield further information on the biological differences between neuroblastoma cells and foetal neuroblasts.

As the antigen defined by KP-NAC8 is present on neoplastic neuroblasts but not on normal foetal neuroblasts, it is possible that the antigen might be a differentiation-

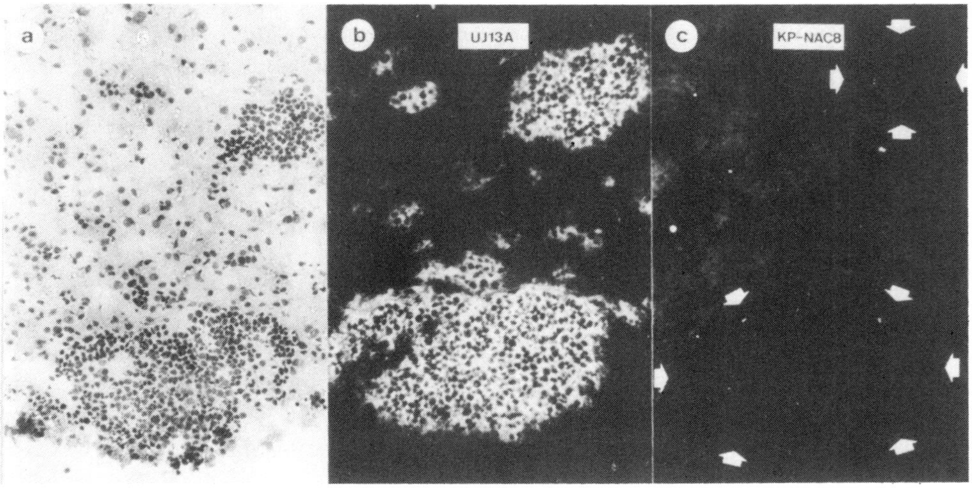

Fig. 5 — Photomicrographs of foetal neuroblasts in the adrenal gland. Nodular collections of foetal neuroblasts were seen in the medulla. a, May–Giemsa staining; b,c, indirect immunofluorescence with UJ13A (b) and KP-NAC8 (c). Foetal neuroblasts in nodular collections were stained with UJ13A (b), but not with KP-NAC8 (encircled with arrows) (c).

related antigen that is selectively expressed on neuroblastoma cells. In addition, since the same antigen is present on ganglion cells but not on Schwann cells in ganglioneuroma tissue and foetal sympathetic ganglion, it might be related in the same manner to the direction of the differentiation pathway of neuroblasts to ganglion cells. This antigen was resolved to be an $M \approx 200\,000$ cell surface protein on neuroblastoma cells. The characterization of the biological and biochemical nature of the antigen defined by KP-NAC8 is of great interest for neuroblastoma research. Further characterization of antigens of foetal neuroblasts will contribute to a greater understanding of the biological nature of neuroblastoma and is our next goal to be resolved.

ACKNOWLEDGEMENTS

We gratefully thank Dr. J. T. Kemshead, Dr. A. A. Green, Dr. L. Helson, Dr. J. Minowada, Dr. C. P. Reynolds, Dr. R. C. Seeger, Dr. K. Sagawa, Dr. T. J. Triche, Dr. H. Koprowski and Dr. A. H. Ross for kindly providing either cell lines or monoclonal antibodies. We are very indebted to Ms. Yumi Kamada for secretarial assistance.

This work was supported in part by grants for cancer research from the Ministry of Health and Welfare and from the Ministry of Education (No. 59480236) of Japan.

REFERENCES

[1] Reynolds, C. P., Smith, R. G. & Frenkel, E. P. (1981). The diagnostic dilemma of the "small round cell neoplasm": catecholamine fluorescence and tissue culture morphology as markers for neuroblastoma. *Cancer* **48** 2088–2094

[2] Triche, T. J. & Askin, F. B. (1983). Neuroblastoma and the differential diagnosis of small-, round-, blue-cell tumors. *Human Pathol.* **14** 569–595
[3] Triche, T. J. (1986) Neuroblastoma — biology confronts nosology. *Arch. Pathol. Lab. Med.* **110** 994–997
[4] Reynolds, C. P. & Smith, R. G. (1982). Diagnostic and biologic markers for neuroblastoma. In: C. Pochedly (ed.) *Neuroblastoma: Clinical and Biological Manifestations*, Elsevier, New York, pp. 131–167
[5] Seeger, R. C. (1982). Immunology of neuroblastoma. In: C. Pochedly (ed.), *Neuroblastoma: Clinical and Biological Manifestations*, Elsevier, New York, pp. 169–182
[6] Berthold, F. (1984). Monoclonal antibodies to human neuroblastoma cells and other solid tumors. In: R. H. Kennett, K. H. Bechtol & T. J. McKearn (eds.) *Monoclonal Antibodies and Functional Cell Lines*, Plenum, New York, pp. 215–238
[7] Kemshead, J. T. (1984). Monoclonal antibodies to neuroblastoma antigens. In: G. W. Wright (ed.) *Monoclonal Antibodies and Cancer*, Dekker, New York, pp. 49–80
[8] Kemshead, J. T., Fritschy, J., Asser, U., Sutherland, R. & Greaves, M. F. (1982). Monoclonal antibodies defining markers with apparent selectivity for particular haematopoietic cell types may also detect antigens on cells of neural crest origin. *Hybridoma* **1** 109–123
[9] Kemshead, J. T. & Coakham, H. B. (1983). The use of monoclonal antibodies for the diagnosis of intracranial malignancies and the small round cell tumours of childhood. *J. Pathol.* **141** 249–257
[10] Sugimoto, T., Tatsumi, E., Kemshead, J. T., Helson, L., Green, A. A. & Minowada, J. (1984). Determination of cell surface membrane antigens common to both human neuroblastoma and leukemia–lymphoma cell lines by a panel of 38 monoclonal antibodies. *J. Natl. Cancer Inst.* **73** 51–57
[11] Sugimoto, T., Sawada, T., Arakawa, S., Matsumura, T., Sakamoto, I., Takeuchi, Y., Reynolds, C. P., Kemshead, J. T. & Helson, L. (1985). Possible differential diagnosis of neuroblastoma from rhabdomyosarcoma and Ewing's sarcoma by using a panel of monoclonal antibodies. *Jpn. J. Cancer Res. (Gann.)* **76** 301–307
[12] Donner, L., Triche, T. J., Israel, M. A., Seeger, R. C. & Reynolds, C. P. (1985). A panel of monoclonal antibodies which discriminate neuroblastoma from Ewing's sarcoma, rhabdomyosarcoma, neuroepithelioma, and hematopoietic malignancies. In: A. E. Evans, G. J. D'Angio & R. C. Seeger (eds.) *Advances in Neuroblastoma Research*, Alan R. Liss, New York, pp. 347–366
[13] Oppedal, B. R., Brandtzaeg, P. & Kemshead, J. T. (1987). Immunohistochemical differentiation of neuroblastoma from other small round cell neoplasms of childhood using a panel of mono- and polyclonal antibodies. *Histopathol.* **11** 363–374
[14] Kennett, R. H. & Gilbert, F. (1979). Hybrid myelomas producing antibodies against a human neuroblastoma antigen present on fetal brain. *Science* **203** 1120–1121
[15] Seeger, R. C., Dannon, Y. L., Zeltzer, P. M., Maidman, J. E. & Rayner, S. A. (1980). Expression of fetal antigens by human neuroblastoma cells. In:

A. E. Evans (ed.) *Advances in Neuroblastoma Research*, Raven Press, New York, pp. 199–207.

[16] Kemshead, J. T., Bickneel, D. & Greaves, M. F. (1981). A monoclonal antibody detecting an antigen shared by neural and granulocytic cells. *Pediatr. Res.* **15** 1282–1286

[17] Reynolds, C. P. & Smith, R. G. (1982). A sensitive immunoassay for human neuroblastoma cells. In: M. S. Mitchell & H. F. Oettgen (eds.) *Hybridoma in Cancer Diagnosis and Treatment*, Raven Press, New York, pp. 235–240

[18] Cheung, N.-K. V., Saarinen, U. M., Neely, J. E., Landmeier, B., Donovan, D. & Coccia, P. F. (1985). Monoclonal antibodies to a glycolipid antigen on human neuroblastoma cells. *Cancer Res.* **45** 2642–2649

[19] Frantz, C. N., Duerst, R. E., Ryan, D. H., Gelsomino, N. L., Constine, L. S. & Gregory, P. K. (1985). Anti-neuroblastoma monoclonal antibodies which do not bind to bone marrow cells. In: A. E. Evans, G. J. D'Angio & R. C. Seeger, (eds.) *Advances in Neuroblastoma Research*, Alan R. Liss, New York, pp. 485–499

[20] Frantz, C. N., Duerst, R. E., Ryan, D. H., Constine, L. S., Gelsomino, N., Rust, L. & Gregory, P. (1986). A monoclonal anti-neuroblastoma antibody that discriminates between human nonhematopoietic and hematopoietic cell types. *Hybridoma* **5** 297–306

[21] Rettig, W. J., Chesa, P. G., Jennings, M. T., Spengler, B. A., Melamed, M. R., Oettgen, H. F., Biedler, J. L. & Old, L. J. (1985). Cell surface antigen of human neuroblastoma is related to nuclear antigen of normal cells. *Proc. Natl. Acad. Sci. USA* **82** 6894–6899

[22] Rettig, W. J., Dracopoli, N. C., Chesa, P. G., Spengler, B. A., Beresford, H. R., Davies, P., Biedler, J. L. & Old, L. J. (1985). Role of human chromosome 11 in determining surface antigenic phenotype of normal and malignant cells. *J. Exp. Med.* **162** 1603–1619

[23] Schonmann, S. M., Iyer, J., Laeng, H., Gerber, H. A., Kaser, H. & Blaser, K. (1986). Production and characterization of monoclonal antibodies against human neuroblastoma. *Int. J. Cancer* **37** 255–262

[24] Mujoo, K., Spiro, R. C. & Reisfeld, R. A. (1986). Characterization of a unique glycoprotein antigen expressed on the surface of human neuroblastoma cells. *J. Biol. Chem.* **261** 10299–10305

[25] Gross, N., Beck, D., Carrel, S. & Munoz, M. (1986). Highly selective recognition of human neuroblastoma cells by mouse monoclonal antibody to a cytoplasmic antigen. *Cancer Res.* **46** 2988–2994

[26] Mujoo, K., Cheresh, D. A., Yang, H. M. & Reisfeld, R. A. (1987). Disialoganglioside GD2 on human neuroblastoma cells: target antigen for monoclonal antibody-mediated cytolysis and suppression of tumor growth. *Cancer Res.* **47** 1098–1104

[27] Matsumura, T., Sugimoto, T., Sawada, T., Saida, T. & Kemshead, J. T. (1988). Distinctive membrane phenotypes of neuroblastoma cells and fetal neuroblasts by a panel of monoclonal antibodies. In: A. E. Evans, G. J. D'Angio, & R. C. Seeger (eds.) *Advances in Neuroblastoma Research*, Alan R. Liss, New York, in press.

[28] Matsumura, T., Sugimoto, T., Sawada, T., Amagai, T., Negoro, S. &

Kemshead, J. T. (1987). Cell surface membrane antigen present on neuroblastoma cells but not fetal neuroblasts recognized by a monoclonal antibody (KP-NAC8). *Cancer Res.* **47** 2924–2930
[29] Schnegg, J. F., Diserens, A. C., Carrel, S., Accolla, K. S. & de Tribolet, N. (1981). Human glioma-associated antigens detected by monoclonal antibodies. *Cancer Res.* **41** 1209–1213
[30] De Muralt, B., de Tribolet, N., Diserens, A. C., Carrel, S. & Mach, J. P. (1983). Reactivity of antiglioma monoclonal antibodies for a large panel of cultured gliomas and other neuroectoderm derived tumors. *Anticancer Res.* **3** 1–6
[31] Carrel, S., de Tribolet, N. & Mach, J. P. (1982). Expression of neuroectodermal antigens common to melanomas, gliomas, and neuroblastomas I. Identification by monoclonal anti-melanoma and anti-glioma antibodies. *Acta Neuropathol (Berl.)* **57** 158–164
[32] Bourdon, M. A., Wikstrand, C. J., Furthmayr, H., Matthews, T. J. & Bigner, D. D. (1983). Human glioma–mesenchymal extracellular matrix antigen defined by monoclonal antibody. *Cancer Res.* **43** 2796–2805
[33] Wikstrand, C. J., Bigner, S. H. & Bigner, D. D. (1984). Characterization of three restricted specificity monoclonal antibodies raised against the human glioma cell line D-54MG. *J. Neuroimmunol.* **6** 169–186
[34] Cairncross, J. G., Mattes, M. J., Beresford, H. R., Albino, A. P., Houghton, A. N., Lloyd, K. O. & Old, L. J. (1982). Cell surface antigens of human astrocytoma defined by mouse monoclonal antibodies: identification of astrocytoma subsets. *Proc. Natl. Acad. Sci. USA* **79** 5641–5645
[35] Liao, S.-K., Clarke, B. J., Kwong, P. C., Brickenden, A., Gallie, B. L. & Dent, P. B. (1981). Common neuroectodermal antigens on human melanoma, neuroblastoma, retinoblastoma, glioblastoma and fetal brain revealed by hybridoma antibodies raised against melanoma cells. *Eur. J. Immunol.* **11** 450–454
[36] Seeger, R. C., Rosenblatt, H. M., Imai, K. & Ferrone, S. (1981). Common antigenic determinants on human melanoma, glioma, neuroblastoma, and sarcoma cells defined with monoclonal antibodies. *Cancer Res.* **41** 2714–2717
[37] Saxton, R. E., Mann, B. D., Morton, D. L. & Burk, M. W. (1982). Monoclonal antibodies to 125 kd and 95 kd proteins on human melanoma cells: comparison with other monoclonal-defined melanoma antigens. *Hybridoma* **1** 433
[38] Irie, R. F., Sze, L. L. & Saxton, R. E. (1982). Human antibody to OFA-I, a tumour antigen, produced *in vitro* by Epstein–Barr virus-transformed human B-lymphoid cell lines. *Proc. Natl. Acad. Sci. USA* **79** 5666–5670
[39] Cahan, L. D., Irie, R. F., Singh, R., Cassidenti, A. & Paulson, J. C. (1982). Identification of a human neuroectodermal tumor antigen (OFA-I-2) as ganglioside GD2. *Proc. Natl. Acad. Sci. USA* **79** 7629–7933
[40] Ross, A. H., Grob, P., Bothwell, M., Elder, D. E., Ernst, C. S., Marano, N., Ghrist, B. F. O., Slemp, C. C., Herlyn, M., Atkinson, B. & Koprowski, H. (1984). Characterization of nerve growth factor receptor in neural crest tumors using monoclonal antibodies. *Proc. Natl. Acad. Sci. USA* **81** 6681–6685
[41] Helson, L., Weinberger, C., Helson, C. & Lieberman, P. (1984). Neuroectodermal tumor and monoclonal antibodies. *Amer. J. Pediatr. Hematol. Oncol.* **6** 227–231

[42] Eisenbarth, G. S., Walsh, F. S. & Nirenberg, M. (1979). Monoclonal antibody to plasma membrane antigen of neurons. *Proc. Natl. Acad. Sci. USA* **76** 4913–4917
[43] Kemshead, J. T., Ritter, M. A., Cotmore, S. F. & Greaves, M. F. (1982). Human Thy-1: expression on the cell surface of neuronal and glial cells. *Brain Res.* **236** 451–461
[44] Seeger, R. C., Danon, Y. L., Rayner, S. A. & Hoover, F. (1982). Definition of a Thy-1 determinant on human neuroblastoma, glioma, sarcoma and teratoma cells with a monoclonal antibody. *J. Immunol.* **128**, 983–989
[45] Kemshead, J. T., Fritschy, J., Garson, J. A., Allan, P., Coakham, H., Brown, S. & Asser, U. (1983) Monoclonal antibody UJ127:11 detects a 220,000–240,000 kda. glycoprotein present on a sub-set of neuroectodermally derived cells. *Int. J. Cancer.* **31** 187–195
[46] Allan, P. A., Garson, J. A., Harper, E. I., Asser, U., Coakham, H. B., Brownell, B. & Kemshead, J. T. (1983). Biological characterization and clinical application of a monoclonal antibody recognizing an antigen restricted to neuroectodermal tissue. *Int. J. Cancer* **31** 591–598
[47] Kemshead, J. T., Fritschy, J., Asser, U., Sutherland, R. & Greaves, M. F. (1982). Monoclonal antibodies defining markers with apparent selectivity for particular haematopoietic cell types may also detect antigens on cells of neural crest origin. *Hybridoma* **1** 109–123
[48] Wikstrand, C. J., Bourdon, M. A., Pegram, C. N. & Bigner, D. D. (1982). Human fetal brain antigen expression common to tumors of neuroectodermal tissue origin. *J. Neuroimmunol.* **3** 43–62
[49] Wikstrand, C. J. & Bigner, D. D. (1982). Expression of human fetal brain antigens by human tumors of neuroectodermal origin as defined by monoclonal antibodies. *Cancer Res.* **42** 267–275
[50] McMichael, A. J., Pilch, J. R., Galfre, G., Manson, D. Y., Fabre, J. W. & Milstein, C., (1979). A human thymocyte antigen defined by a hybrid myeloma monoclonal antibody. *Eur. J. Immunol.* **9** 205–210
[51] Reinherz, E. L., Kung, P. C., Goldstein, G., Levey, R. H. & Schlossman, S. F. (1980). Discrete stages of human intrathymic differentiation: analysis of normal thymocytes and leukemic lymphoblasts of T-cell lineage. *Proc. Natl. Acad. Sci. USA* **77** 1588–1592
[52] Abramson, C. S., Kersey, J. H. & LeBien, T. W. (1981). A monoclonal antibody (BA-1) reactive with cells of human B lymphocyte lineage. *J. Immunol.* **126** 83–88
[53] Kersey, J. H., LeBien, T. W., Abramson, C. S., Newman, R., Sutherland, R. & Greaves, M. (1981). p24: a human leukemia associated and lymphohemopoietic progenitor cell surface structure identified with monoclonal antibody. *J. Exp. Med.* **153** 726–731
[54] Lipinski, M., Braham, K., Caillaud, J-M., Carlu, C. & Tursz, T. (1983). HNK-1 antibody detects an antigen expressed on neuroectodermal cells. *J. Exp. Med.* **158** 1775–1780
[55] Boucheix, C., Perrot, J. Y., Mirshani, M., Fournier, N., Billard, M., Bernadou, A. & Rosenfeld, C. (1982). Monoclonal antibodies against acute lymphoblastic leukemia differentiation antigens (meeting abstract). In: *First Inter-*

national Workshop of Human Leukocyte Differentiation Antigens, Hospital Saint-Louis, Paris, p. AP-4
[56] Kodama, Y., Peiper, S. C., Melvin, S. L., Metzger, D. W., Tarnowski, B. H. & Green, A. A. (1983). A monoclonal antibody (SJ-9A4) to p24 present on common ALLs, neuroblastomas and platelets 1. Characterization and development of a unique radioimmunometric assay. *Leukemia Res.* **7** 487–498
[57] Lampson, L. A., Fisher, C. A. & Whelan, J. P. (1983). Striking paucity of HLA-A,B,C and B2-microglobulin on human neuroblastoma cell lines. *J. Immunol.* **130**, 2471–2478
[58] Gibson, F. M. & Kemshead, J. T. (1987). A monoclonal antibody (FMG25) that can differentiate neuroblastoma from other small round-cell tumors of childhood. *Int. J. Cancer.* **39** 554–559
[59] Cuttitta, F., Rosen, S., Gazdar, A. F. & Minna, J. D. (1981). Monoclonal antibodies that demonstrate specificity for several types of human lung cancer. *Proc. Natl. Acad. Sci. USA* **78** 4591–4595
[60] De Leiy, L., Poppema, S., Nulend, J. K., ter Haar, A., Schwander, E., Ebbens, F., Postmus, P. E & The, T. H. (1985). Neuroendocrine differentiation antigen on human lung carcinoma and Kulchitski cell. *Cancer Res.* **45** 2192–2200
[61] Kemshead, J. T. (1988). A multi centre blind study on the reactivity of a panel of monoclonal antibodies on neuroblastoma and other small round cell tumours of childhood. In: A. E. Evans, G. J. D'Angio, & R. C. Seeger (eds.) Alan R. Liss, New York, in press
[62] Seeger, R. C. (1982). Neuroblastoma: clinical perspectives, monoclonal antibodies, and retinoic acid. *Ann. Intern. Med.* **97** 873–884
[63] Reynolds, C. P., Biedler, J. L., Spengler, B. A., Reynolds, D. A., Ross, R. A., Frenkel, E. P. & Smith, R. G. (1986). Characterization of human neuroblastoma cell lines established before and after therapy. *J. Natl. Cancer Inst.* **76** 375–387
[64] Kodama, Y., Azuma, E., Kamiya, H. & Sakurai, M. (1986). Phenotype profile of human neuroblastoma cell lines: association with morphological characteristics. *Br. J. Cancer* **54** 711–715
[65] Rettig, W. J., Spengler, B. A., Chesa, P. G., Old, L. J. & Biedler, J. L. (1987). Coordinate changes in neuronal phenotype and surface antigen expression in human neuroblastoma cell variants. *Cancer Res.* **47** 1383–1389
[66] Sugimoto, T., Sawada, T., Negoro, S., Kidowaki, T., Morioka, H., Matsumura, T., Kemshead, J. T. and Seeger, R. C. C. (1985). Altered expression of cell surface membrane antigens in a common acute lymphoblastic leukemia antigen-expressing neuroblastoma cell line (SJ-N-CG) with morphological differentiation. *Cancer Res.* **45** 358–364
[67] Reynolds, C. P. & Maples, J. (1985) Modulation of cell surface antigens accompanies morphological differentiation of human neuroblastoma cell lines. In: A. E. Evans, G. J. D'Angio & R. C. Seeger (eds.) *Advances in Neuroblastoma Research*, Alan R. Liss, New York, pp. 13–37
[68] Gross, N., Beck, D., Favre, S. & Carrel, S. (1987). *In vitro* antigenic modulation of human neuroblastoma cells induced by IFN-γ, retinoic acid and dibutyryl cyclic AMP. *Int. J. Cancer* **7** 521–529

5

Neuroblastoma: chromosome abnormalities and their possible significance

Fred Gilbert and **Subal Chattopadhyay**
Departments of Pediatrics, Obstetrics and Gynecology and Reproductive Science,
Mount Sinai School of Medicine,
New York, NY 10029, USA

1. INTRODUCTION

In 1960, Nowell and Hungerford reported the first association between a specific chromosome abnormality, termed the Philadelphia chromosome, and a particular human cancer, chronic myelogenous leukaemia [1]. With the introduction of chromosome banding techniques in the 1970s, it became apparent that the Philadelphia chromosome was not a deleted G-group chromosome, as originally postulated, but a reciprocal translocation between chromosome 22 and another autosome (non-sex chromosome), most commonly number 9 [2]. In the years following, consistent or recurrent chromosome abnormalities have been described in many human malignancies, predominantly leukaemias and lymphomas [3,4].

The number of solid tumours in which cytogenetic analysis has identified consistent chromosome rearrangements is small, the result of basic difficulties in preparing karyotypes, as well as in establishing cell lines in culture from such tissues. Neuroblastoma is an exception: a category of solid tumour from which multiple, independent permanent cell lines have been derived and from which karyotypes have been prepared, both from primary tumours and cultured cell lines. This has led, over the last several years, to the accumulation of a considerable body of data on the cytogenetics of neuroblastoma. In a 1984 review, we summarized the results from our laboratory and those published by other investigators to that point [5]. A recent literature search, bringing these data up to date as of the end of 1987, is summarized in Table 1.

2. CHROMOSOME 1

The single chromosome most frequently involved in structural and numerical abnormalities in neuroblastoma is number 1. The abnormalities are of two major

Table 1 — Chromosome abnormalities in human neuroblastomas karyotyped prior to 1984 [5] and subsequently [49–58]

(A)

Series	Total	Chromosome abnormalities: $1p^-$	+1q	+17q	HSR–DMS
1984	35	25 (71%)	13 (37%)	8 (23%)	23 (66%)
1984–1987	30	17 (57%)	1 (3%)	4 (13%)	27 (90%)

(B)

Series	Direct–line	Chromosome abnormalities: Total	$1p^-$	HSR–DMs
1984	D	22	18	6
	L	14	9	12
	Total	36	27 (75%)	18 (50%)
1984–1987	D	63	39	35
	L	23	14	22
	Total	86	53 (62%)	57 (66%)
	Overall total	122	80 (66%)	75 (62%)

(C)

Series–chromo. abnormality	Tumour stage: I	II	III	IV	NS	Total
1984–1987						
$1p^-$	2 (33%)	1 (17%)	8 (80%)	30 (70%)	12	53 (62%)
No $1p^-$	4	5	2	13	8	32
HSR–DMs	1 (20%)	1 (13%)	5 (42%)	35 (73%)	13	55 (62%)
No HSR–DMs	5	8	7	13	1	34

(A) Summary of abnormalities in complete karyotypes from tumours and cell lines in both series.
(B) Summary of analyses for chromosome 1p markers and HSR–DMs in direct preparations and karyotypes from cultured cell lines in both series.
(C) Comparison of abnormalities of 1p and HSR–DMs in individual tumour stages in cases described 1984–1987 (staging as per [26]; NS=not specified).
1p: deletion–rearrangements of chromosome 1p, +1q, +17q=extra whole chromosomes or long area segments.

types: deletions or rearrangements resulting in the loss of structural material from the short arm (1p) and additional whole chromosomes or long arm (1q) segments. The majority of 1p marker chromosomes represent unbalanced translocations in which the chromosomes of origin of the segments transposed to 1p are unknown. This has made it difficult to define the precise breakpoints on 1p in different tumours or cell lines. Published reports have described breaks at bands 1p21, 1p22, 1p31, and 1p32 in the marker 1p chromosomes in individual neuroblastomas. The consensus from the cases published to date is that the marker chromosomes 1 of neuroblastoma

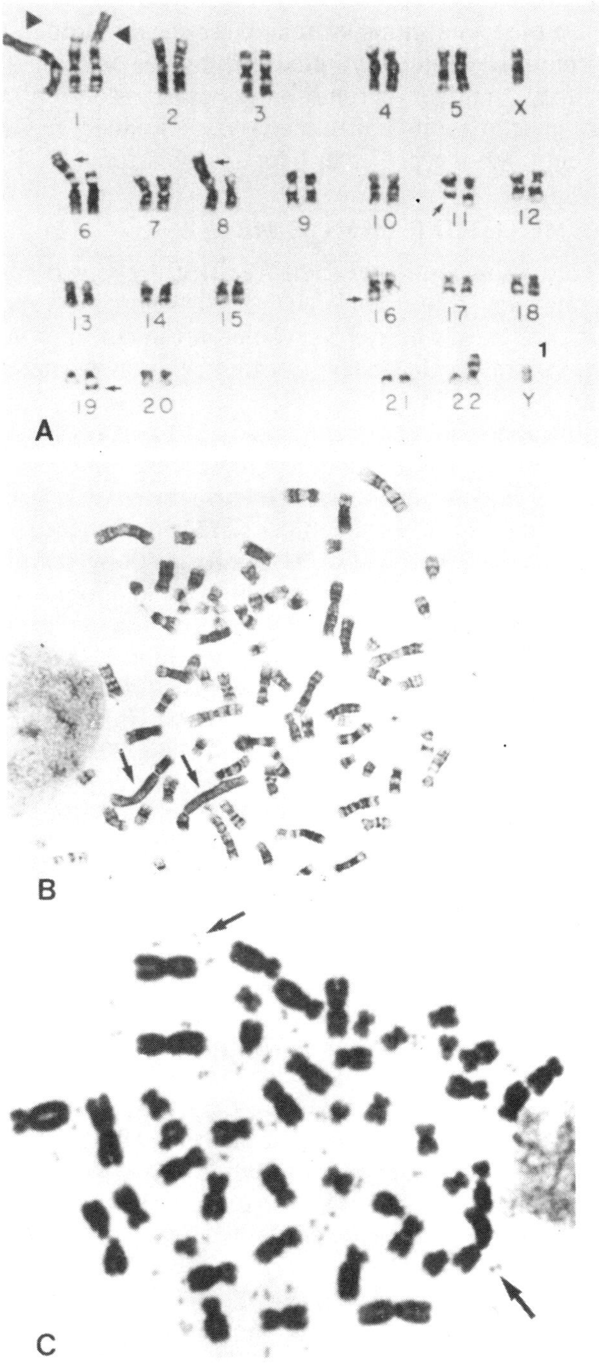

Fig. 1 — (A) Abnormal chromosome 1p in neuroblastoma (example). Karyotype of an IMR.5 subclone containing three chromosomes 1 per cell. Middle number 1 is normal; two outer chromosomes 1 have HSR originating at 1p31. (B) Arrow to homogenously staining region (HSR) in G-banded metaphase. (C) Arrow to DMs in conventionally stained (non-banded) metaphase.

consistently involve the loss of transposition of sequences distal to band 1p32.

The extra 1q material frequently noted can involve additional whole chromosomes, additional $1p^-$ marker chromosomes, or translocated segments of 1q. However, the presence of additional 1q material is a frequent finding in karyotypes from many different tumour types other than neuroblastoma [3,6].

3. CHROMOSOMES OTHER THAN NUMBER 1

Chromosome 17 has also been found to be frequently involved in abnormalities of number and organization in neuroblastoma. The abnormalities result in additional 17q material, either as extra whole chromosomes 17 or iso(17q). As with the more common extra 1q, extra 17q has been reported as an associated finding in other tumour types [3,6].

Data concerning abnormalities of chromosomes 1 and 17, as well as of homogeneously staining regions and double minutes (described below), are summarized in Table 1. Differences evident in the relative frequencies of individual cytogenetic abnormalities in neuroblastoma between the series prior to, and after, 1984 presumably reflect an artifact of selection. For Table 1A only those karyotypes from which information about all of the common abnormalities could be obtained were included; when only information about $1p^-$ and HSR, double minute chromosomes (DMs) was available (Table 1B), the number of tumours included in the updated series was increased and the overall frequency of $1p^-$ markers was 70%, as in the earlier series.

Structural and numerical abnormalities involving virtually all of the autosomes have been noted in individual neuroblastomas (Table 2). The majority of these reports identify changes unique to single cases. However, our recent update discloses the preferential involvement of distal 11q in deletions, translocations, and as the site of insertion of a homogeneously staining region (HSR) (Table 3).

The focus on 11q is interesting because of the previous report of a constitutional (that is, present in every cell in the body) chromosomal change in a family with neuroblastomas in multiple individuals in different generations [7,8]. A father had two children with documented neuroblastoma by different wives. One affected child had died prior to being karyotyped, but the father, the presumed carrier of a gene change predisposing to neuroblastoma, and a living child affected were found to share a constitutional chromosome change: an 'atypical' chromosome 11, subsequently shown to be an inversion, inv(11) (q21–q23) [9]. The initial excitement surrounding this finding and the speculation that the identified segment included a gene change involved in neuroblast transformation decreased somewhat when it was reported that one of the father's children who did not carry the variant 11 had a child with neuroblastoma [8]. The possibility of meiotic recombinations separating the 11q inversion from a possible gene on the same chromosome involved in tumorigenesis exists, however. Although concordant segregation of neuroblastoma with the variant 11 in this family could not be proved, interest in chromosome 11 as the site of a neuroblastoma gene locus persists.

4. HOMOGENEOUSLY STAINING REGIONS AND DOUBLE MINUTES

In 1976, Biedler and Spengler described a novel cytogenetic abnormality, the HSR, in karyotypes from a Chinese hamster ovary (CHO) cell line and from a human

Table 2 — Chromosome abnormalities in human neuroblastomas

Chromosome number	Numerical abnormalities	HSR	Structural abnormalities
1	+1	1p	del(1p13);del(p22);del(1p32);t(1;9)(q11;p11);t(1;9)(q22;p24);t(1;14)(p32;q31);t(1;11)(?;p?);t(1;?)(p32;?)
2			$2q^+$
3	−3		t(3;15)(q13;q26)
4	−4;+4		$4p^+$;del(4q31)
5		5q	
6	+6	6q	$6p^+$;$6q^+$;del(6q23);del(6q25)
7	−7;+7	7p	$7p^+$;$7q^-$;del(7q22);t(7;11)(q36;q13);t(7;16)(q22;q24)
8			t(8;?)(q24;?)
9			$9q^+$;t(1;9)(q11;p11);t(1;9)(q22;q24);t(9;15)(p11;p11)
10			$10q^+$;del(10q22)
11			$11p^+$;$11q^-$;del(11q23);t(1;11)(p?;p?);t(7;11)(q36;q13)
12			$12q^+$
13		13p	$13p^+$;$13q^+$;t(13;18)(p11;q11)
14	+14		t(1;14)(p32;q31)
15	−15;+15		t(9;15)(p11;p11)
16		16p	$16q^+$;t(7;16)(q22;q24)
17			17^+;del(17p11)
18	−18;+18		$18p^+$;t(13;18)(p11;q11)
19	+19		$19q^+$
20	+20		$20q^+$
21	−21		
22	−22		$22p^+$;$22q^+$;del(22q13)

Chromosome abnormalities as catalogued in [3]. Chromosome number=individual chromosomes in karyotype. Numerical abnormalities=consistent deviations from diploid number. HSR=site of origin of HSR. Structural abnormalities=deletions and rearrangements involving individual chromosomes (nomenclature as per [59]).

neuroblastoma line [10]. The HSR is a chromosome segment generally longer than any single band in the standard karyotype. It also stains with intermediate intensity over its entire length; it does not show the alternating pattern of dark and light (or dull and bright) bands that characterizes the rest of the karyotype. The HSR shares the staining properties of another cytogenetic anomaly, the so-called DMs. The latter are paired chromatin bodies without centromeres. They vary in size and number within and between tumours and cell lines. The DMs are maintained in dividing cell populations by attaching to the ends of chromosomes as they separate at mitosis.

We were able to confirm the existence of HSRs, and of DMs, in neuroblastomas, in both primary tumours and cell lines [11], and subsequently, to document how common they were in this tumour type [5]. We were also able to show that, in somatic cell hybrids, the breakdown or disappearance of an HSR from a cell could be associated with the appearance of DMs [12]. In cell lines containing both HSR and DMs, the general rule is that an individual cell will contain one or the other anomaly, not both. However, single cells with both have been described [13].

Taken together, these observations indicate that the HSR and DMs are alternate

Table 3 — Abnormalities of chromosome 11q in human neuroblastomas

Case	Chromosome 11q abnormality	Reference
IMR-5	del(11) (q223→qter)	[13]
SW-083	HSR(11) (q23)	[54]
MH-078	HSR(11) (q25)	[54]
SS-104	t(11;?) (q25;?)	[54]
CHP382	t(4;11) (q28;q23)	[49]
SMS-KANR	t(11;?) (q23;?)	[56]
SMS-SAN	t(11;17) (q24;q21)	[56]
Patient 68	t(11;?) (q21;?)	[58]
LA-N-2	HSR(11) (q24)	[60]
Patient NBB	t(7;11) (q36;q13)	[61]
Patient NJF	del(11) (q23→qter)	[61]

Structural abnormalities involving chromosome 11 in tumour cell karyotypes of individual cases. Nomenclature as per [59].

manifestations of the same biological phenomenon. The functional significance of the HSR was suggested by their discovery in a line of CHO cells that was resistant to the drug methotrexate and known to contain multiple copies of a gene conferring drug resistance, i.e. for dihydrofolate reductase [10]. It was proposed, and subsequently proved (by *in situ* hybridization of radiolabelled probes to metaphase spreads), that the HSR in this particular cell line is the site of amplification of the gene for dihydrofolate reductase.

However, the majority of neuroblastomas reported to contain HSR and/or DMs are from untreated patients, and no evidence for the amplification of drug resistant-genes in any primary tumours has been found. Because amplification of members of a recently described category of genes, the cellular homologues of retroviral oncogenes (the so-called c-onc genes), had been noted in other cancers, DNAs from HSR-containing neuroblastomas were screened with molecular probes specific for different viral oncogenes (v-onc) and c-onc genes. All of the neuroblastomas so studied were found to contain multiple copies (from 10 to over 500 copies) of a gene resembling the cellular homologue of v-myc (the oncogene associated with avian myelocytomatosis virus) [14,15]. The new gene was designated N-myc, to distinguish it from c-myc, and mapped to band 2p23; c-myc had previously been assigned to 8q24 [16,17].

Amplification of one or more different oncogenes has been noted in individual examples of virtually every tumour type. For most cancers, the particular oncogene(s) amplified in any one tumour appear to be non-specific [18]. Neuroblastoma is, to date, the only cancer in which amplification uniformly involves the same oncogene. (Apparent exceptions — a subset of round cell tumours in children containing multiple copies of c-myc — have been reclassified as 'peripheral neuroepitheliomas', because they share a specific chromosome rearrangement, t(11,22) [19].)

The amplification unit (amplicon) in different neuroblastomas can include sequences other than N-myc, both expressed (that is, transcribed as messenger RNAs) and unexpressed [20,21]. All of the sequences contained within the amplicons are derived from chromosome 2. They are not, however, necessarily contiguous on the chromosome of origin; co-amplified sequences in individual neuroblastomas have been mapped to different regions of bands 2p1 and 2p2, a chromosome segment extending over several million base pairs of DNA [21]. Neither are they fixed in position within the amplicon; the precise pattern of sequences and their organization within the amplicon can be different in different neuroblastomas [21].

The size of the amplicon has been estimated in different neuroblastoma cell lines by different methods. Using light and electron microscopic measurements and comparisons of HSRs with normal chromosome segments, estimates of amplicon size of between 1.5×10^6 and 9.8×10^6 bp of DNA have been produced [22,23]. Using an in-gel hybridization technique, estimates of $(2.8–4.0)\times10^5$ bp of DNA have been generated [24].

The HSRs in neuroblastoma always develop at sites in the karyotype distinct from 2p23, the band to which N-myc has been mapped. Translocation is, therefore, a necessary step (prerequisite?) for visible amplification. While it appears likely that rearrangement of sequences within and between amplicons can occur as the HSR develops and increases in length *in situ,* the mechanisms responsible for the initial development of the amplicon are unclear. Does, for example, rearrangement of sequences ultimately included within the amplicon occur on 2p prior to translocation (perhaps, by analogy with the molecular rearrangements that develop within the immunoglobulin gene complexes on chromosomes 2,14, and 22 in B-cells), or does rearrangement occur only extrachromosomally in DMs, or in the HSR after integration into the chromosome? Does the original amplicon develop on chromosome 2 by a form of anomalous replication (speculations about mechanisms of replication are presented in [25]), then fall off to become a DM that can insert into a chromosome and develop as an HSR? Alternatively, a rearranged segment from chromosome 2 may translocate–integrate into another chromosome directly, developing as an HSR, which is, in turn, unstable and can break down to be released as DMs or continue to reduplicate *in situ.* Studies to distinguish between these possibilities are ongoing.

5. CLINICAL STAGES OF NEUROBLASTOMA

Neuroblastoma has been subdivided into five clinically distinguishable stages, based on patterns of involvement with disease and the age at which the tumour is discovered [26]. Stage I constitutes disease limited to the site of origin (most commonly, the adrenal medulla). Stage II includes cases with local spread of tumour, but not across the midline. Stage III designates regional spread, crossing the midline. Stage IV comprises patients with widespread metastatic disease to distant sites, such as lymph nodes, bone or lung. Stage IV-S, the rarest form, is limited to patients under one year of age at diagnosis, in whom disease is limited to primary site, liver, skin, and/or bone marrow, but never involving bone (as with stage IV).

The prognosis is worst for stage IV disease and best for stages I, II, and IV-S. Most significant, perhaps, is the frequent association of IV-S with spontaneous regression. In over 85% of IV-S cases, many of which have very extensive involvement with tumour, primarily as massive hepatomegaly, the disease will completely disappear, over months to years from the time of original diagnosis, without any therapeutic intervention. Some 15% of cases, however, progress to stage IV.

6. CYTOGENETIC ABNORMALITIES, STAGE, DISEASE PROGRESSION, AND DIAGNOSIS

Some studies have related particular cytogenetic changes to disease progression and prognosis in neuroblastoma. In a case report comparing karyotypes obtained from a primary tumour, originally classified as stage III, with those obtained from multiple metastases 11 months later, two significant changes were noted: a change in chromosome number per cell, from multiple modes with a peak near tetraploidy, in the original sample, to a single, near-diploid mode in all metastases; an increase in the number of chromosomes 1 per cell, from two in the initial tumour samples to three in all metastases, two of which were $1p^-$ markers (resulting, effectively, in additional 1q material in each cell) [27].

In a study relating karyotypic abnormalities to stage, the authors concluded that significant aneuploidy — near-triploid modes — in the absence of $1p^-$ and N-myc amplification is associated with local, limited disease, and near diploidy is associated with more advanced disease [28]. Of 30 cases reviewed, 14 were near diploid and all were in stages III and IV. Of those with the poorest prognosis, the 8 cases classified as stages I or II, 7 were triploid and 1 was tetraploid.

Two studies utilizing flow cytometry to measure DNA content as an index to ploidy came to similar conclusions. In one, the tumour cells from 6 of 10 stage IV neuroblastomas were near diploid, while significant aneuploidy (approaching tetraploidy) was evident in the tumour cells from 23 of 25 patients in all other stages [29]. Included in the latter group were four stage IV-S tumours: all were near triploid, with a DNA content peak at 1.5 vs. 1.0 for normal, diploid cells. Of 17 patients with significant aneuploidy for whom follow-up data were available, all demonstrated responsiveness (complete or partial remissions) to a course of a standard chemotherapeutic protocol; 6 patients whose tumours exhibited near-diploid modes did not respond to the same protocol (although 4 did respond to a different protocol).

In a second study, significant aneuploidy (approaching or exceeding tetraploidy) and a low percentage of tumour cells in the S, G_2, and M phases of the cell cycle were associated with prolonged survival (at least 2 years) [30]. Significant aneuploidy was seen in the tumour cells from 63% of survivors, compared with only 21% of non-survivors. Of the tumours from patients that were classified as stages III or IV, 14 had near-diploid modes; of the tumours from 18 patients in stages I, II, or IV-S, 10 were aneuploid.

We have also published the results of the chromosome analyses of primary tumours, skin nodules, and/or bone marrow aspirates from four patients with stage IV-S disease [31]. In all patients, significant aneuploidy developed or was evident in cells collected at the time of tumour regression.

Deletion–translocation marker chromosomes 1 (those resulting in the loss of material from 1p) tend to occur more commonly in stages III and IV than in the localized stages I and II (in approximately 70% of the former, and 20% of the latter; Table 1C). The advanced, more severe stages of neuroblastoma have also been associated with the presence of HSR and/or DMs in tumour cell karyotypes, as well as N-myc amplification [32]. Data from a series of recent case reports are summarized in Table 1C. More than 70% of tumours of stage IV contain HSR–DMs and amplified N-myc, whereas the comparable figure for stages I and II is generally less than 20%.

One can conclude, then, that neuroblastomas with a generally good prognosis tend to be significantly aneuploid and to lack the $1p^-$ marker and HSR–DMs (or evidence of N-myc amplification). Those tumours with the poorest prognosis (predominantly, stage IV), tend to contain near-diploid modes, one or more $1p^-$ markers, and HSR–DMs.

7. A UNIFYING HYPOTHESIS RELATING CHROMOSOME ABNORMALITIES TO THE DEVELOPMENT OF NEUROBLASTOMA

The existence of familial recurrences of neuroblastoma and the fact that familial cases often involve multiple, distinct primary tumours (in one or both adrenals), and are identified at significantly younger ages than are the sporadic cases, led Knudson to propose the 'two hit' hypothesis some years ago [33]. This argues that at least two gene changes are necessary for neuroblastoma tumorigenesis: one can be inherited or develop spontaneously in the somatic target cell, a neuroblast, but only those neuroblasts in which a second specific mutation event also occurs will become transformed.

The patterns of recurrence in two other childhood solid tumours, retinoblastoma and Wilms' tumour, are also consistent with the 'two hit' hypothesis [34]. However, unlike neuroblastoma, each of these cancers has also been associated with a constitutional chromosomal change. Retinoblastoma occurs in a subgroup of patients with the 13q deletion syndrome: in all of those in whom the deletion includes band 13q14 [35]. Wilms' tumour occurs in association with aniridia (absence of the iris in the eye) and constitutional deletions of band p13 in chromosome 11 [36].

It is not unreasonable to postulate that a chromosome abnormality unique to a particular tumour type will point to the site of a gene contributing to (or responsible for) malignant transformation. Accepting this premise, then, would mean that a deletion at 13q14 may constitute a 'first hit' in retinoblastoma. If this is the case, the 'second hit' could result from the loss of activity of the homologous allele at band q14 on the other member of the pair of chromosomes 13. Evidence supporting this hypothesis, utilizing recombinant DNA probes that detect polymorphic sequences on chromosome 13 and make it possible to distinguish between the two chromosomes 13 in a cell, has been presented [37]. The conclusion from this work is that the homozygous loss of activity of a gene at 13q14 (through deletion, mutation, or chromosome loss) is a prerequisite for retinoblast transformation.

A number of investigators have taken advantage of the development of probes specific for polymorphic sequences on every chromosome to extend the search for genes responsible for tumorigenesis to other human cancers. By comparing the patterns of retention or loss of sequences unique to individual chromosomes in tumour vs. constitutional tissue (e.g. white blood cells, fibroblasts) from the same patients, it has been possible to associate the loss of sequences on chromosomes 2,5,11,13, and 22 with the development of uveal melanoma, colon cancer, Wilms' tumour, certain breast cancers, and meningioma respectively [38–42]. The fact that the homozygous loss of activity of single genes has been demonstrated in several different cancers raises the possibility that a similar mechanism contributes to the development of many, if not all, cancers in man.

The search for the chromosomal site of the gene responsible for tumorigenesis in neuroblastoma has long focused on the distal short arm of chromosome 1, the segment most commonly involved in structural rearrangements in this cancer (Table 1). Establishing that a particular chromosome segment does indeed contain such a gene requires that the loss of DNA sequences from that chromosome be confined to the tumour; determining that the loss involves DNA sequences requires that the chromosomes in question be structurally intact (at the light microscopic level) in the tumour. Unfortunately, comparison of the retention or loss of chromosome-1p-specific DNA sequences in neuroblastoma vs. constitutional tissue from the same patients has proved difficult for two reasons: the majority of published karyotyped cases are from patients that are no longer alive, making it impossible to obtain normal constitutional tissue for comparison, and the newly diagnosed and karyotyped cases from whom sufficient tumour and constitutional tissues can be obtained for DNA analysis are predominantly stage IV and involve tumours already carrying a $1p^-$ deletion–rearrangement.

The emphasis on chromosome 1 has, therefore, shifted to the isolation of transcriptionally active sequences from chromosome-1-enriched gene libraries. If a gene on chromosome 1 were involved in tumorigenesis, its transcribed product, an mRNA, would presumably be absent or altered in neuroblastoma, but present in mature cells of the peripheral nervous system, and possibly in other normal cells as well. Studies using a similar approach were recently successful in identifying a gene on chromosome 13 as the putative retinoblastoma locus [43].

Other investigators have begun to look for the loss of sequences on chromosomes other than number 1, particularly those identified as the sites of rare deletions in tumour cell karyotypes (Table 2). Among the latter are del(11q23), del(17p11), and del(22q13). The first band is included in the constitutional inversion in one family with recurrent neuroblastomas described previously [9] and is adjacent to one breakpoint in the reciprocal translocation that characterizes the histologically similar peripheral neuro-epithelioma ((11;22) (q24:q12) [19]); 17p11 is the site of a gene responsible for the development of one form of neurofibromatosis (NF) [44], and 22q13 is at or near the site of a gene responsible for the development of a second form of NF [45]. A possible association between neuroblastoma and NF, an autosomal dominant inherited disorder, is intriguing, because NF results in benign and malignant tumours derived from cells of neural crest origin, the same tissue from which neuroblastoma develops. Also, neuroblastomas have been reported in patients with NF at a frequency higher than that in the general population.

In addition to gene changes that are presumed to play primary roles in tumorigenesis, another category of gene changes is postulated to contribute to tumour progression: the ability of a tumour to expand and spread in the host [46]. The number of chromosome abnormalities per cell is known to increase when tumours are sampled at different times in a single patient's illness; this is particularly well described in leukaemias and lymphomas [47]. The chromosome changes that develop and accumulate in the course of a tumour's evolution are non-random but are also not unique to the individual tumour types in which they occur. The description of extra 1q, extra 17q, and HSR–DMs with amplification of single oncogenes in neuroblastomas, for example, is not specific or unique to this cancer. As noted previously, each of these findings has been reported in examples of different tumour types. However, these abnormalities tend to be associated with more severe forms of the cancers in which they have been described, as with neuroblastoma. This is consistent with the hypothesis that they play a secondary role in tumour progression.

Having said that there are gene changes responsible for tumorigenesis and for tumour progression, we now must elaborate a genetic scheme that will take into account these findings, as well as the postulates of the 'two-hit' hypothesis and the phenomena of tumour regression and neuroblastoma *in situ*. Tumour regression has already been discussed in the context of stage IV-S disease; neuroblastoma *in situ* refers to the finding, in some 10% of autopsies of infants who died for reasons other than cancer, of localized foci of neuroblastoma-like cells in the adrenal medulla [48]. As the frequency of neuroblastoma *in situ* is so much higher than that of neuroblastoma itself (only 1 in 10 000–20 000 infants, or less), it must be assumed that most neuroblastoma *in situ* foci regress or mature to more benign, differentiated cell types (e.g. ganglioneuroma).

We can postulate that neuronal differentiation involves the passage of the neural crest cell through several, as-yet undefined, steps, leading to final maturation as a neuron in either the central or the peripheral nervous systems (the latter includes the adrenal medulla and spinal ganglia, primary sites for neuroblastoma development). We further postulate that the transition between individual steps in the neuronal lineage is controlled by single genes and that the homozygous loss of activity of such genes through mutations, deletions, etc. leads to a block to further passage through the lineage. The blocked cell will continue to divide to produce a localized focus of neuroblasts, recognized as neuroblastoma *in situ* or neuroblastoma, stage IV-S. (Neural crest derivatives are widely dispersed throughout the organism giving rise to disparate cell types, including melanocytes in skin; presumably, rests of neural crest cells in skin give rise to the skin nodules in IV-S.)

With successive divisions of cells in these foci, two outcomes are possible: an abnormal segregation of chromosomes at mitosis, producing significant aneuploidy, or an accumulation of additional gene changes in near-diploid cells. Significant aneuploidy is likely to be a pre-terminal event: cells die, slow in their division rate, or stop dividing entirely. Cell death could account for the tumour regression in IV-S disease; cessation of division, with expression of the differentiated phenotype, could account for the maturation seen in ganglioneuroma; and a slowing in cell division rate might result in the localized tumours seen in stage I and II neuroblastomas (triploidy and tetraploidy have already been associated with stage I and II disease [28,29]).

The accumulation of a limited number of additional gene changes, if they occur in a cell that is diploid or near diploid in mode, further enchances its growth potential, resulting in stage III disease. Metastatic spread, the hallmark of stage IV, presumably requires still more gene changes, particularly those resulting from extra 1q chromosomes, extra 17q chromosomes, and the development of HSR–DMs.

In this scheme, the 'two-hit' hypothesis is modified to a 'two-step' hypothesis, requiring two different genetic steps, both likely to involve homozygosity at distinct loci, for full tumorigenesis. Homozygosity, as a prerequisite for 'step one', is suggested by the transformation of only some neuroblasts in familial cases, even though all cells carry the predisposing first gene change. Homozygosity, as a requirement for 'step two', is likely because of the relative rarity of neuroblastoma, as compared with the frequency of neuroblastoma *in situ*.

One of the required 'two steps' is likely to involve a gene on distal 1p; the site of the other gene change is, at present, unknown. The homozygous involvement of a gene on 1 p is most likely responsible for the second step, as the description of $1p^-$ markers is highest in neuroblastoma stages III and IV (the finding of this change in a small percentage of stage I and II tumours, presumably reflects the fraction of cases that will go on to stage III or IV diseases).

If the scheme presented is correct, the identification of the genes involved, and of the changes associated with each, in neuroblastoma, will provide additional criteria for classification, as well as for determining prognosis and the need for therapy in individual cases. It could also lead to the identification of individuals at risk of developing neuroblastoma in familial cases. The biochemical characterization of such genes may also provide insight into more effective approaches to therapy.

ACKNOWLEDGEMENT

This work was supported by a grant from the National Institutes of Health (CA 41759).

REFERENCES

[1] Nowell, P. C. & Hungerford, D. A. (1960). A minute chromosome in human chronic granulocytic leukemia. *Science* **132** 1497

[2] Rowley, J. D. (1977). A new consistent chromosomal abnormality in chronic myelogenous leukemia identified by quinacrine fluorescence and Giemsa staining. *Nature* **243** 290–293

[3] Mittelman, F. (1983). Catalogue of chromosome aberrations in cancer. *Cytogenet. Cell Genet.* **36** 9–515

[4] Yunis, J. J. (1986). Chromosomal rearrangements, genes, and fragile sites in cancer. In: V. DeVita, S. Hellman & S. Rosenberg (eds.) *Important Advances in Oncology — 1986,* Lippincott, Philadelphia, pp. 93–128

[5] Gilbert, F., Feder, M., Balaban, G., Brangman, D., Lurie, D. K., Podolsky, R., Rinaldt, V., Vinikoor, N. & Weisband, J. (1984). Human neuroblastomas and abnormalities of chromosomes 1 and 17. *Cancer Res.* **44** 5444–5449

[6] Rowley, J. D. (1977). Mapping of human chromosomal regions related to neoplasia. Evidence from chromosomes 1 and 17. *Proc. Natl. Acad. Sci. USA* **74** 5729–5733

[7] Pegelow, C., Ebbin, A. J., Powars, D. & Towner, J. (1975). Familial neuroblastoma. *J. Pediatr.* **87** 763–765

[8] Hecht, F. & Kaiser-McGaw, B. (1981). Chromosomes in familial neuroblastoma. *J. Pediatr.* **98** 334

[9] Hecht, F., Hecht, B. K., Northrup, J. C., Trachtenberg, N., Wood, T. S. &

Cohen, J. D. (1982). Genetics of familial neuroblastoma: long range studies. *Canc. Genet. Cytogenet.* **7** 227–230

[10] Biedler, J. L. & Spengler, B. A. (1976). Metaphase chromosome anomaly: association with drug resistance and cell-specific products. *Science* **191** 185–187

[11] Balaban-Malenbaum, G. & Gilbert, F. (1977). Double minute chromosomes and their relationship to the homogeneously staining regions in chromosomes of a human neuroblastoma cell line. *Science* **198** 739–741

[12] Balaban-Malenbaum, G. & Gilbert, F. (1980). The proposed origin of double minutes from HSR-marker chromosomes in human neuroblastoma hybrid cell lines. *Canc. Genet. Cytogenet.* **2** 239–248

[13] Balaban-Malenbaum, G. & Gilbert, F. (1980). Relationship between homogeneously staining regions and double minute chromosomes in human neuroblastoma cell lines. In: A. Evans (ed.) *Advances in Neuroblastoma Research,* Raven Press, New York, pp. 97–107

[14] Kohl, N. E., Kanda, N., Schreck, R. R., Bruns, G., Latt, S. A., Gilbert, F. & Alt, F. (1983). Transposition and amplification of oncogene-related sequences in human neuroblastoma. *Cell* **35** 359–367

[15] Schwab, M., Alitalo, K., Klemphauer, K.-H., Varmus, H. E., Bishop, J. M., Gilbert, F., Brodeur. G., Goldstein, M. & Trent, J. (1983). Amplified DNA domain with limited homology to the *myc* cellular oncogene is shared by human neuroblastoma cell lines and a human neuroblastoma tumor. *Nature* **305** 245–248

[16] Schwab, M., Varmus, H. E., Bishop, J. M., Grzeschik, K.-H., Naylor, S., Sakageuchi, A., Brodeur, G. & Trent, J. (1984). Chromosome localization in normal human cells and neuroblastoma of a gene related to *c-myc. Nature* **308** 288–291

[17] Neel, B. G., Jhanwar, S. C., Chaganti, R. S. & Hayward, W. (1982). Two human *c-onc* genes are treated on the long arm of chromosome 8. *Proc. Natl. Acad. Sci. USA* **79** 7842–7846

[18] Slamon, D. J., deKernion, J. B., Verma, I. M. & Clive, M. J. (1984). Expression of cellular oncogenes in human malignancies. *Science* **224** 256–262

[19] Whang-Peng, J., Triche, T. J., Knutsen, T., Miser, J., Douglass, E. C. & Israel, M. Chromosome translation in peripheral neuroepithelioma. *N. Engl. J. Med.* **311** 584–585

[20] Kohl, N. E., Gee, C. E. & Alt, F. (1985). Activated expression of the *N-myc* gene in human neuroblastomas and related tumors. *Science* **226** 1335–1337

[21] Shiloh, Y., Korf, B., Kohl, N. E., Sakai, K., Brodeur, G., Harris, P., Kanda, N., Seeger, R. C., Alt, F. & Latt, S. A. (1986). Amplification and rearrangement of DNA sequences from the chromosomal region of 2p24 in human neuroblastomas. *Canc. Res.* **46** 5297–5301

[22] Brodeur, G. & Seeger, R. C. (1986). Gene amplification in human neuroblastomas: basic mechanisms and clinical implications. *Canc. Genet. Cytogenet.* **19** 101–111

[23] Garson, J. A., van den Berghe, J. A. & Kemshead, J. T. (1987). High-resolution in site hybridization technique using biotinylated NMYC oncogene probe reveals periodic structure of HSRs in human neuroblastoma. *Cytogenet. Cell Genet.* **45** 10–15

[24] Kinzler, K. W., Zehnbauer, B. A., Brodeur, G. M., Seeger, R. C., Trent, J. M., Meltzer, P. S. & Vogelstein, B. (1986). Amplification units containing human N-myc and C-myc genes. *Proc. Natl. Acad. Sci. USA* **83** 1031–1035

[25] Schimke, R. T., Brown, P. C., Kaufman, R. J., McGrogan, M. & Slate, D. L. (1980). Chromosomal and extrachromosomal localization of amplified dihydrofolate reductase genes in cultured mammalian cells. *Symp. Quant. Biol. Cold Spring Harbor* **45** 785–797

[26] Evans, A. E., D'Angelo, G. & Randolph, J. (1971). A proposed staging for children with neuroblastoma. *Cancer* **27** 374–378

[27] Feder, M. & Gilbert, F. (1983). Clonal evolution in a human neuroblastoma. *J. Nat. Canc. Inst.* **70** 1051–1056

[28] Kaneko, Y., Kanda, N., Maseko, N., Sakurai, M., Tsuchida, Y., Tokeda, T., Okabe, I. & Sakurai, M. (1987). Different karyotypic patterns in early and advanced stage neuroblastomas. *Canc. Res.* **47** 311–318

[29] Look, A. T., Hayes, F. A., Nitschke, R., McWilliams, N. & Green, A. (1984). Cellular DNA content as a predictor of response to chemotherapy in infants with unresectable neuroblastoma. *N. Engl. J. Med.* **311** 231–235

[30] Gansler, T., Chatten, J., Varello, M., Bunin, G. & Atkinson, B. (1986). Flow cytometric DNA analysis of neuroblastoma. *Cancer* **58** 2453–2458

[31] Balaban, G. & Gilbert, F. (1983). Neuroblastoma IV-S: chromosome analysis. *N. Engl. J. Med.* **309** 989

[32] Brodeur, G. M., Seeger, R. C., Schwab, M., Varmus, H. E. & Bishop, J. M. (1984). Amplification of N-myc in untreated human neuroblastomas correlates with advanced disease stage. *Science* **224** 1121–1124

[33] Knudson, A. G. & Strong, L. C. (1972). Mutation and cancer: neuroblastoma and pheochromocytoma. *Am. J. Hum. Genet.* **24** 514–532

[34] Knudson, A. G. (1976). Genetics and the etiology of childhood cancer. *Ped. Res.* **10** 513–517

[35] Yunis, J. J. & Ramsay, N. (1978). Retinoblastoma and subband deletion of chromosome 13. *Am. J. Dis. Child.* **132** 161–163

[36] Riccardi, V. M., Sujansky, E., Smith, A. C. & Francke, U. (1978). Chromosomal imbalance in the aniridia–Wilms' tumor association. *Pediatrics* **61** 604–610

[37] Cavenee, W. K., Dryja, T. P., Phillips, R. A., Benedict, W. F., Godbout, R., Gallee, B. L., Murphree, A. L., Strong, L. C. & White, R. L. (1983). Expression of recessive alleles by chromosomal mechanisms in retinoblastoma. *Nature* **305** 779–784

[38] Makai, S. & Dryja, T. P. (1986). Loss of alleles at polymorphic loci on chromosome 2 in ureal melanoma. *Canc. Genet. Cytogenet.* **22** 45–53

[39] Solomon, E., Voss, R., Hall, V., Bodmer, W. F., Jass, J. R., Jeffreys, A. J., Lucibello, F. C., Patel, I. & Rider, S. H. (1987). Chromosome 5 allele loss in human colorectal carcinomas. *Nature* **328** 616–619

[40] Koufos, A., Hansen, M. F., Copeland, N. G., Jenkins, N. A., Lampkin, B. C. & Cavenee, W. K. (1985). Loss of heterozygosity in three embryonal tumors suggests a common pathogenetic mechanism. *Nature* **316** 330–334

[41] Lundberg, C., Skoog, L., Cavenee, W. K. & Nordenskjold, M. (1987). Loss of heterozygosity in human ductal breast tumors indicates a recessive mutation on chromosome 13. *Proc. Natl. Acad. Sci. USA* **84** 2372–2376

[42] Seizinger, B. R., De La Monte, S., Atkins, L., Gusella, J. F. & Martuza, R. (1987). Molecular genetic approach to human meningioma: loss of genes on chromosome 22. *Proc. Natl. Acad. Sci. USA* **84** 5419–5423
[43] Friend, S. H., Bernards, R., Rogelj, S., Weinberg, R. A., Rapaport, J. M. & Dryja, T. P. (1986). A human DNA segment with properties of the gene that predisposes to retinoblastoma and osteosarcoma. *Nature* **323** 643–646
[44] Barker, D., Wright, C., Nguyen, K., Cannon, L., Fain, P., Goldgar, D., Bishop, D. T., Carey, J., Baty, B., Kivlin, J., Willard, H., Waye, J. S., Greig, G., Leinwand, L., Nakamura, Y., O'Connell, P., Leppert, M., Lalouel, J.-M., White, R. & Scolnick, M. (1987). Gene for von Recklinghausen neurofibromatosis is in the pericentromeric region of chromosome 17. *Science* **236** 1100–1102
[45] Rouleau, G. A., Wertelecki, W., Haines, J., Hobbs, W., Trofatter, J., Seizinger, B., Martuza, R., Superneua, D., Conneally, P. M. & Gusella, J. F. (1987). Genetic linkage of bilateral acoustic neurofibromatosis to a DNA marker on chromosome 22. *Nature* **329** 246–248
[46] Gilbert, F. (1983). Chromosomes, genes, and cancer: a classification of chromosome abnormalities in cancer. *J. Natl. Canc. Inst.* **71** 1107–1114
[47] Nowell, P. C. (1976). The clonal evolution of tumor cell populations. *Science* **194** 23–28
[48] Beckwith, J. B. & Perria, E. V. (1963). In situ neuroblastomas: a contribution to the natural history of neural crest tumours. *Am. J. Pathol.* **43** 1089–1100
[49] Emanuel, B., Balaban, G., Boyd, J., Grossman, A., Negishi, M., Parmiter, A. & Glick, M. C. (1985). N-myc amplification in multiple homogeneously staining regions in two human neuroblastomas. *Proc. Natl. Acad. Sci. USA* **82** 3736–3740
[50] Franke, F., Forster, W., Rudolph, B. & Lampert, F. (1985). Metastatic neuroblastoma in an infant. *Eur. J. Pediatr.* **143** 305–308
[51] Hafez, M., El-Meadday, M., Sheir, M., Al-Tonbarry, Y., Nada, N. & El-Desoky, I. (1985). Chromosomal analysis of neuroblastoma. *Br. J. Canc.* **51** 237–243
[52] Kaneko, Y., Tsuchida, Y., Maseki, N., Takasaki, N., Sakurai, M. & Saito, S. (1985). Chromosome findings in human neuroblastomas xenografted in nude mice. *Jpn. J. Canc. Res.* **76** 359–364
[53] Robson, J. A. & Sidell, N. (1985). Ultrastructural features of a human neuroblastoma cell line treated with retinoic acid. *Neuroscience* **14** 1149–1162
[54] Franke, F., Rudolph, B., Christiansen, H., Harbott, J. & Lampert, F. (1986). Tumor karyotype may be important in the prognosis of human neuroblastoma. *J. Canc. Res. Clin. Oncol.* **111** 266–272
[55] Franke, F., Rudolph, B. & Lampert, F. (1986). Translocation (19;?) in two stage II neuroblastomas. *Canc. Genet. Cytogenet.* **20** 129–135
[56] Reynolds, C. P., Biedler, J. L., Spengler, B. A., Reynolds, D. A., Ross, R. A., Frenkel, E. P. & Smith, R. G. (1986). Characterization of human neuroblastoma cell lines established before and after therapy. *J. Natl. Canc. Inst.* **76** 375–387
[57] Christiansen, H., Franke, F., Bartram, C. R., Adolph, S., Rudolph, B., Harbott, J., Reiter, A. & Lampert, F. (1987). Evolution of tumor cytogenetic aberrations and N-myc oncogene amplification in a case of disseminated

neuroblastoma. *Canc. Genet. Cytogenet.* **26** 235–244
[58] Kaneko, Y., Kanda, N., Maseki, N., Sakurai, M., Tsuchida, Y., Taheda, T., Okabe, I. & Sakurai, M. (1987). Different karyotypic patterns in early and advanced state neuroblastomas. *Canc. Res.* **47** 311–318
[59] Bergsma, D. (1978). Human chromosome nomenclature. *Cytogenet. Cell Genet.* **21** 312–409
[60] Biedler, J., Ross, R., Shanske, S. & Spengler, B. (1980). Human neuroblastoma cytogenetics. In: A. Evans (ed.) *Advances in Neuroblastoma Research,* Raven Press, New York, pp. 81–96
[61] Brodeur, G., Green, A., Hayes, F. A., Williams, K., Williams, D. & Tsiatis, A. (1981). Cytogenetic features of human neuroblastomas and cell lines. *Canc. Res.* **41** 4678–4686

6

Modulation of neuroblastoma growth by biological factors and pharmacological agents

Bernard Mirkin,
Departments of Pediatrics and Pharmacology, Director, Division of Clinical Pharmacology, University of Minnesota Health Sciences Center, Box 87, UMHC, Minneapolis, MN 55455, USA; and
Donald W. Fink, Jr.,
NIGMS/NICHD, Section on Growth Factors, National Institutes of Health, Bethesda, MD 20892, USA

1. INTRODUCTION

Perhaps the most enigmatic characteristic of neuroblastoma tumours has been their propensity to undergo seemingly capricious changes in growth and maturation. Clearly, the extent to which a primitive neuroblast differentiates is an extremely variable process since local rests of immature cells can be found as *in situ* tumours in children under three months of age. Histopathological data suggest their incidence to be between 1:179 and 1:259, a frequency that is 40 times the projected rate of occurrence. Neuroblastoma tumours are detected in approximately one per 10 000 live-born infants; hence one must inevitably conclude that spontaneous regression or further differentiation of *in situ* neuroblastoma is a common phenomenon, occurring in at least 1% to 2% of all cases [1].

The ensuing discussion will focus on endogenous and exogenous factors that modulate neuroblastoma cell replication, biological maturation and tumorigenicity with emphasis on the mechanisms by which different modalities may exert their actions. The murine neuroblastoma (MNB) model and, wherever possible, data obtained from studies of human neuroblastoma will be utilized to define the respective influence(s) of these factors on tumour biology. Previous investigations have revealed significant similarities in the basic characteristics of murine and human neuroblastoma, suggesting this comparative approach to be both relevant and valid [2].

2. FACTORS REGULATING NEUROBLASTOMA GROWTH AND DIFFERENTIATION

The rate of proliferation and stage of differentiation achieved by neuroblastoma cells appears to be determined by factors that can be categorized as either endogenous or exogenous in nature. Among the endogenous factors that appear to be of major significance and which will be considered in this review are host age and biological maturation, tissue innervation (somatic and autonomic), polypeptide growth factors, oncogenes and cellular receptors.

2.1 Endogenous factors

2.1.1 Influence of host age and biological maturation

The interval between inoculation of MNB tumour cells and detection of a palpable mass (tumour onset time) has been shown to be influenced by both host age and tumour load [3]. Recent studies have demonstrated a small, but statistically significant, increase in tumour onset time following MNB tumour implantation in 14- and 21-day-old mice when compared with 7- and 56-day-old animals. Differences in MNB tumour incidence and growth rate that are host-age related have been proposed from *in situ* studies using adult and neonatal mice [4]. In contrast to adult animals, neonatal mice inoculated with an identical number of MNB tumour cells either failed to develop tumours or had a marked reduction in the number of tumours developed. Recent studies in our laboratory, however, have not been able to confirm a reduced rate of tumour growth or incidence in 24-h-old neonatal mice inoculated with either 10^4 or 10^6 MNB cells [3].

While the precise influence of host age on MNB tumour growth remains to be resolved, this parameter does appear to influence biochemical differentiation as defined by tumour cell catecholamine profile. The synthesis and degradation of catecholamines by MNB tumours *in situ* [5] and in tissue culture [6,7] has been demonstrated. The presence of both dopamine and norepinephrine suggests some partial differentiation along the adrenergic pathway, a process that has been shown to parallel the induction of MNB cell maturation in tissue culture [8]. Since gene product expression of catecholamine synthesizing enzymes and their neurohormonal transmitters in the primordial neuroblast is highly regulated, an elevation of MNB tumour catecholamine content *in situ* might also be predicted in association with an increment in synthetic enzyme activity and advancing degrees of cellular differentiation.

Insofar as the effect of host age on this process is concerned, the analysis of catecholamine concentrations in tumours obtained from animals implanted with MNB cells at 7, 14, 21 and 56 days of age did not reveal any significant differences [3]. It is of interest that the tumours of mice implanted with MNB cells at 1 day of age had significantly lower epinephrine and dopamine concentrations than older animals. These results suggest that host age may play a role in regulating the biochemical differentiation of MNB *in situ* during the early post-natal period, since the effect is no longer present 7 days post-natally.

Factors elaborated during embryogenesis and possibly in the early post-natal period modulate and control the differentiation of malignant cells [9]. Some neoplastic cells thought to be non-responsive to normal control mechanisms can be restored to a responsive state during foetal development [10]. Experiments in which embryonal carcinoma cells were injected into mouse blastocysts and subsequently transferred to the uteri of pseudo-pregnant animals demonstrated that neoplastic cells could undergo further differentiation in this environment to form normal embryonic structures. Similar results were reported following placement of MNB cells into the second somite of neurula stage mouse embryos [11,12]. Inoculation of MNB cells into this specific region of the developing embryo resulted in a decreased tumour incidence when that portion of the embryo containing the MNB cells was transplanted into syngeneic host mice.

Since development of the murine neural crest occurs during neurulation, implantation of neural crest derived MNB cells into the neurula stage embryo may permit them to come under regulatory influences that attenuate or eliminate their malignant potential. The limitations of this experimental design make it impossible to determine whether the reduction in tumour incidence occurred because the implanted MNB cells were further differentiated or subject to some cytotoxic action of the embryonic tissue. It is of interest that the response of MNB cells was apparently cell specific, since other types of tumours with different embryological origins were unaffected following implantation into the same somite. The inhibition of MNB growth has also been observed in late stage embryos, suggesting the presence of a generalized regulatory mechanism that is capable of suppressing the growth of all migrating cells until they have reached their appropriate end organ(s) [13].

It has been hypothesized that polypeptides generated and released during active cell growth exert a significant role in both restraining and promoting the morphological differentiation of MNB cells. A substance with these properties has been identified in the culture medium of proliferating glioblasts isolated from the brains of rat foetuses [14]. The growth and DNA synthesis of cultured fibroblasts and glial cell lines were not influenced by this partially purified polypeptide, indicating that the target of this factor may be restricted to replicating neuronal cells, including neuroblastoma. An inverse correlation between the titre of 'neuroblastoma growth inhibitory factor' and host age, if demonstrable, would be consistent with the hypothesis that regulation of neuroblastoma growth and biological maturation of the host are interdependent.

2.1.2 Neurotrophic regulation

2.1.2.1 Somatic nervous system

The 'trophic' influence of the nervous system on normal tissue growth and regeneration has been demonstrated in a variety of studies [15]. In the early 1900s, clinical studies reported that skin tumours did not develop in denervated areas of the epidermis whereas they arose and spread primarily throughout the innervated regions of the skin [16]. More current investigations have clearly demonstrated that tumour growth patterns and mitotic activity may be modified, resulting in either enhancement or inhibition, when functional innervation at the site of tumour implantation is absent [17–19]. Of particular interest with respect to neuroblastoma, was the observation that tumour growth rates were reduced following ablation of either the somatic or the sympathetic nervous system.

In 1970, Batkin *et al.* [20] demonstrated that the growth of MNB cells implanted into the gastrocnemious muscle of mice was transiently inhibited following peripheral section of the sciatic nerve. This was associated with histological changes in cell morphology characterized by a reduction in nuclear size and shape. Subsequent studies by this group confirmed their original findings and further demonstrated that denervation decreased mitotic activity in implanted MNB cells [21]. These data implied that neurotrophic factors associated with somatic motor (and possibly sensory) nerves exerted a growth-enhancing effect on MNB tumours only when a functional neuro-effector system existed.

2.1.2.2 Sympathetic nervous system

During the past decade, strong evidence supporting the role of the autonomic nervous system, in particular its adrenergic component, as a modulator of MNB growth has been established. This concept is of particular significance since it suggests that ganglia and neurons, which are terminally differentiated neural structures deriving from the same embryonic anlage as neuroblastoma, can exert a regulatory effect on neoplastic cells.

The early observations of Angeletti and Levi-Montalcini demonstrated that treatment of adult MNB tumour-bearing mice with 6-hydroxydopamine (6-OHDA) inhibited *in situ* tumour growth [18]. This response was attributed to a direct effect of 6-OHDA on the MNB tumour since it was administered at the time of MNB cell implantation and during the period of tumour growth. In retrospect, these results may have been too narrowly interpreted owing to the restriction of the experimental design, which did not allow discrimination between the neurolytic effects of 6-OHDA on adrenergic nerve terminals and its direct cytotoxic action on MNB cells. Thus, the possibility that sympathetic denervation produced by 6-OHDA might also contribute to the suppression of tumour growth still remained a viable option. Other investigators following this lead treated adult mice with 6-OHDA to produce a post-ganglionic adrenergic sympathectomy prior to implantation of MNB cells [22]. The growth of MNB tumours in sympathectomized adult mice was shown to be significantly slower and tumour size smaller than in control mice.

Recently, the relationship between host age, sympathetic nervous system ablation and MNB tumour growth has been re-evaluated [23]. These studies demonstrated an increase in tumour onset time following implantation of MNB cells into sympathectomized adult mice. However, tumour growth rate after initial palpation was similar to that of vehicle-treated adult animals. In contrast, sympathectomy of neonatal mice caused a significantly greater increase in tumour onset time and also decreased tumour growth rate when MNB cells were implanted into mice one month after neonatal sympathectomy.

It is important to emphasize that the decrease in MNB tumour growth observed in mice sympathectomized as neonates did not result in a prolonged survival time. If malignant potential is defined in terms of the relationship between tumour size at the time of host death and the number of days animals survived after MNB tumour cell implantation, then neonatal sympathectomy appears to have enhanced the malignancy of MNB even though tumour growth rate was inhibited. This conclusion is based on the finding that sympathectomized mice developed smaller tumours but survived the same number of days (post-tumour implantation) as control animals, even though the latter had significantly larger tumours at death (Fink and Mirkin, unpublished data).

Development of the blood–brain barrier in mice is not completed until the 7th to 9th post-natal day so that systemically administered 6-OHDA could potentially cross the blood–brain barrier to exert a neurotoxic effect on adrenergic neurons in the central nervous system [24]. Regional reductions in brain norepinephrine have been reported following the systemic injection of 6-OHDA in neonatal animals [25,26]. These data suggest that treatment of neonatal mice with 6-OHDA could have exerted a cytolytic action on central catecholaminergic neurons and thereby an effect on neuroblastoma growth. This site of action would be virtually inaccessible in adult mice owing to the impermeability of their blood–brain barrier to 6-OHDA. The potential relationship between central adrenergic innervation and the age-dependent inhibition of MNB tumour growth produced by 6-OHDA has been investigated by injecting 6-OHDA directly into the central nervous system of neonatal animals [27]. Ablation of central adrenergic neurons decreased MNB tumour growth, although somewhat less than that observed following peripheral sympathectomy. When both central and peripheral adrenergic neurons were ablated, the inhibition of MNB tumour growth produced by the combined intervention exceeded that caused by either central or peripheral sympathectomy alone. These findings suggest that the destruction of central adrenergic neurons in neonatal mice given systemic 6-OHDA is not primarily responsible for the age-dependent differences observed in MNB tumour growth suppression, but that the central and peripheral adrenergic systems exert interactive roles in modulating MNB cell replication.

A trophic influence of the sympathetic ganglion on MNB cell growth has been hypothesized and attributed to the secretion of a mitogenic substance from ganglionic cells. Explants of sympathetic ganglia co-cultured with MNB cells caused an increase in their growth rate [28]. It is of interest that the presence of this 'ganglionic trophic factor' appears to be age dependent. Homogenates prepared from the sympathetic ganglia of newborn rats enhanced the rate of MNB growth in tissue culture, whereas those obtained from adult rats had no effect [29]. These observations demonstrate that neurotrophic growth substances are present in differentiated adrenergic structures and that tissue maturation determines their biological potency. Finally, *in situ* studies have demonstrated that the inhibition of MNB tumour growth caused by neonatal sympathectomy can be reversed by administration of nerve growth factor [23,30].

2.1.3 Nerve growth factors (NGF)

The control of cell replication by endogenously produced polypeptide growth factors has become a major focus of studies on the regulation of malignant transformation [31]. Normal diploid cells grown in the absence of these growth factors do not move through the complete cell cycle and tend to arrest at the G_1–G_0 phase whereas cells that have been mitogenically transformed possess the ability to grow in the absence of such factors. In a simplistic sense, therefore, this single genetically determined characteristic appears to distinguish malignant from normal cells.

The molecular events involved in these processes have been intensively examined and a limited group of genes generally present in normal cells have been defined and designated as proto-oncogenes. The genes were initially identified from studies in which simian sarcoma retrovirus was inoculated into animals, an intervention that led to the rapid induction of malignant fibrosarcomas and glioblastomas [32]. The tumorigenic activity of the retrovirus was found to reside in sequences designated *onc* genes that appear to have been derived from the host genome. Substantial evidence has accumulated to support the view that proto-oncogenes may become active oncogenes by mechanisms other than those involving retroviruses and that they are involved in the naturally occurring transformation of normal to malignant cells.

Of particular significance is recent evidence demonstrating that oncogenes may code for growth factors that are capable of regulating mitogenesis in normal as well as transformed cells. This phenomenon has been demonstrated for platelet-derived growth factor, transforming growth factor and epidermal growth factor. The concept that transformed cells can synthesize, release and respond to their own growth factors was presented as early as 1967 [33]. However, it is only within the past decade that the role of autocrine regulation in cellular function and as a modulator of other mitogenic signals has become widely accepted [34,35].

2.1.3.1 Mitogenic and differentiating actions of NGF

The transition of embryonic neural crest cells into discrete components of the sympathetic nervous system appears to be intimately controlled by NGF. This polypeptide exerts both mitogenic and differentiating actions on neural structures. Hence, it plays a pivotal role in the survival and growth of adrenergic neurons during ontogenesis and probably influences maturation of the neuroblast as well [36,37]. If neuroblastoma constitutes a deviation from the predicted course of adrenergic neuron development, as suggested by its lateral divergence at the stage of neuroblast formation, then NGF could either inhibit neoplastic cell replication by promoting differentiation to a more mature, non-malignant cell form or via its mitogenic action stimulate neuroblastoma cell proliferation (Fig. 1). The inability of neuroblastoma cells to recognize and/or respond appropriately to the signals eliciting the corresponding responses may constitute the primary mechanism that controls the aberrant formation of malignant neuroblastoma from the neuroectoderm.

The medium of MNB tissue cultures contains a growth factor that is biologically similar to NGF isolated from murine submaxillary glands. This substance induced neurite outgrowth from embryonic chick sensory ganglion and was completely blocked by anti-NFG [38,39]. The synthesis and/or release of this growth factor by MNB cells was stimulated by adenosine (in the presence of a phosphodiesterase inhibitor) or prostaglandin E_1. Since both compounds elevate adenylate cyclase activity, the increment in NGF concentration was associated with an elevation in intracellular cyclic AMP levels [39]. Other studies using the C6 glioma cell line have reported an increase in NGF content following activation of β-adrenergic receptors [40,41]. An intriguing observation is that of Furukawa *et al.* [42], who found that catecholamines, such as epinephrine and norepinephrine, increased the NGF content of L-M cells. They postulated that the release of adrenergic neurotransmitter in the synaptic cleft modulates NGF synthesis in the effector cell. This hypothesis

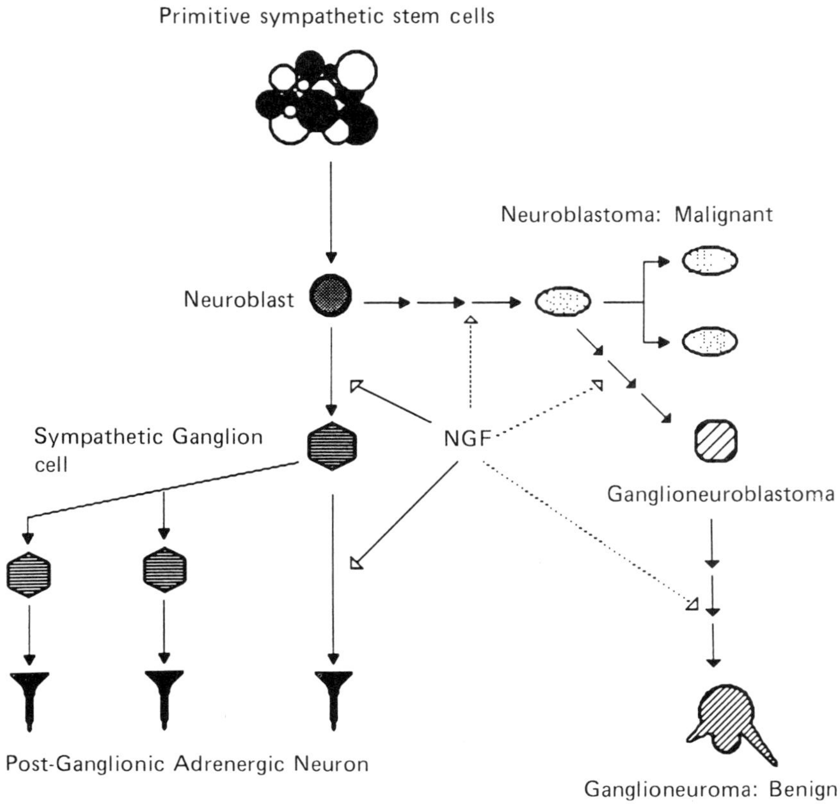

Fig. 1 — Sites of NGF action in neuroectocdermal cell derivatives during oncogenesis.

raises the possibility that the extraneuronal synthesis of NGF which initially sustains the growth and differentiation of adrenergic neurons during embryogenesis may subsequently be regulated by the neuron itself via nerve impulse frequency and quanta of adrenergic neurotransmitter released per nerve impulse. These data suggest a link between β-adrenergic receptor stimulation, adenylate cyclase activation and NGF synthesis.

Adequate evidence confirming the synthesis and secretion of NGF by neuroblastoma cells has been obtained. The effects of NGF on MNB and rat phaeochromocytoma (PC12) cells are quite variable, however, since both mitogenesis and morphological differentiation have been described in each tumour model system. A major experimental problem associated with these studies has been the difficulty in distinguishing between the proliferative and viability–maintaining actions of NGF on neural crest cells [43]. Earlier investigations suggested that NGF stimulated the division of some of its target cells, even though the data did not clearly confirm this hypothesis [44]. The mitogenic action of NGF was clearly demonstrated in MNB clones NB1R and NB6R, cell lines that had previously been shown to bind 2.5S NGF *in vitro* [45]. The NB1R clone, in the presence of NGF, incorporated thymidine into

DNA and underwent cell division whereas the NB6R clone was differentiated further and had a greatly increased survival time in culture.

Rat phaeochromocyte cells (PC12 and variant clonal sublines, U2 and U7) have also been used to discriminate between the seemingly paradoxical mitogenic and differentiating activities of NGF [46]. The variant lines, U2 and U7, were selected because they continue to proliferate actively in the presence of NGF, possess NGF receptors and apparently contain the biological properties necessary to respond to NGF-initiated neurite outgrowth. The reactivity of original PC12 clones differed and they responded by neurite extrusion and a cessation of mitosis.

A variety of human neuroblastoma cell lines, such as clones and LA-N-5 [47] and N5683 [48], extend neurites and undergo differentiation in the presence of NGF, whereas other cell lines, e.g. MC-1XC, CHP-100 and CHP-134, are non-responsive to NGF. The mitogenic and anti-mitogenic responses described above appear to be highly specific for NGF since they are both inhibited by anti-NGF.

2.1.3.2 Cellular receptors

Biological responses in cells sensitive to NGF are elicited via binding of the agonist to specific receptors. There are at least three distinct anatomical regions in NGF-responsive cells that have been shown to possess NGF receptors: the plasma membrane, the nucleus and the synaptic terminals of neurons.

2.1.3.2.1 Plasma membrane receptors. The specific binding of NGF to putative plasma membrane receptors has been observed in a variety of neural crest derivatives including embryonic sympathetic and sensory neurons [49,50] and phaeochromocytoma cells [51,52], as well as murine and human neuroblastoma cells [53,54]. The existence of multiple classes of NGF membrane binding sites was hypothesized by Sutter *et al.* [50] from studies characterizing the binding of radiolabelled β-NGF to cells isolated from the sensory ganglia of 8-day-old chick embryos. Two distinct, saturable NGF-binding sites designated type I (high affinity) and type II (low affinity) with dissociation constants (K_d) of 2.3×10^{-11} M and 1.7×10^{-9} M respectively were identified.

A number of studies describing the kinetics of NGF binding to its receptor have been carried out in the neoplastic, NGF-responsive, rat phaeochromocytoma cell line, PC12. These cells, which have some properties characteristic of adrenal chromaffin cells, respond to NGF by sprouting neurites and undergoing transformation to a sympathetic neuron-like phenotype. In addition to providing generous amounts of homogeneous material for receptor characterization, PC12 cells offer the distinct advantage of not requiring NGF for survival, unlike NGF-responsive neurons. Consequently, PC12 cells and their receptors may be studied and compared both before and after variable periods of exposure to NGF. Utilizing this clonal cell line, the presence of multiple classes of NGF receptor sites was confirmed and they were designated as 'fast' and 'slow' receptors [55]. The 'fast' receptors accounted for 75% of the specific NGF binding measured and were distinguished by their rapid association and dissociation rates. At 37°C the binding of NGF to 'fast' receptors proceeded at a rate that was 5-fold greater than NGF binding to 'slow' receptors, while dissociation of NGF from 'fast' receptors was 40-fold more rapid than from 'slow' receptors. This interpretation contrasted with other investigators who proposed the existence of a homogeneous population of receptors that become heterogeneous following exposure to NGF via a rapid, ligand-induced, conversion from one receptor type to another [56].

The critical issue of receptor heterogeneity, namely whether 'slow' and 'fast' receptors are two distinct proteins or the same protein in two different environments, conformations, or states of chemical modification, has been addressed in the following manner [51]. Plasma membranes that contained primarily 'fast' NGF receptors were prepared from PC12 cells and fused with 3T3 cells lacking receptors. The resultant fused cells were shown to possess NGF receptors, virtually all of which behaved like 'slow' receptors. These studies showed that interconversion of the 'fast' and 'slow' forms of the NGF receptor could occur, but that binding of NGF was not required to mediate conversion from the 'fast' to the 'slow' type. These findings have been confirmed in human neuroblastoma and PC12 cells [54].

The fate of plasma membrane receptors following their interaction with NGF appears to be similar to that of receptors for other polypeptide hormones and growth factors. The receptor–ligand complex undergoes endocytosis and is internalized and degradation of both hormone and receptor in lysosomes may occur. As a consequence of internalization, the number of membrane receptors is decreased or 'down-regulated'. Studies characterizing the binding of NGF to PC12 cells have described an internalization of NGF–receptor complexes that is consistent with the process of endocytosis [57]. The time-dependent decrease in binding of radioactive NGF was associated with degradation of the radioactive ligand and a reduction in the number of surface receptors. Internalization of the receptor–ligand complex appears to be receptor type specific [52]. The 'slow', high-affinity receptors which constitute a minor fraction of the total number of cell surface NGF receptors are endocytosed following binding to NGF, whereas low-affinity. 'fast' receptors remain on the exterior of the plasma membrane after interacting with NGF.

The relationship of high-affinity, 'slow' NGF plasma membrane receptors and cellular response has been studied in mutant PC12 cells that lack high-affinity NGF receptors [58]. Mutant PC12 phaeochromocytoma cell lines, non-responsive to NGF, were selected from mutagen-treated cultures using a double selection procedure in which candidate cultures were identified by their failure to grow neurites in the presence of NGF and to survive in NGF-supplemented serum-free medium. The mutant cultures were also deficient to other NGF-induced responses such as cessation of cell proliferation, changes in glycoprotein composition, induction of ornithine decarboxylase, rapid changes in protein phosphorylation, and cell surface ruffling. In addition to their inability to respond to NGF, the mutant PC12 cell lines could be distinguished from the 'parent' PC12 cells on the basis of two additional features: (1) failure to internalize bound NGF by the normal, saturable, high-affinity mechanism present in 'parent' PC12 cells; (2) the binding of NGF to mutant PC12 cells occurred exclusively at low-affinity sites, whereas 'parent' PC12 cells possessed both high- and low-affinity NGF binding sites. The internalization and response of mutant PC12 cells to epidermal growth factor (EGF) was normal, thus excluding the possibility that a generalized defect in polypeptide hormone processing was responsible for the impaired response of mutant PC12 cells to NGF. These findings led Green and his colleagues to propose the existence of a causal association between the presence of high-affinity, 'slow' NGF receptors, NGF internalization and cellular response [58]. A monoclonal antibody to the 'slow' NGF receptor has been shown to modulate the response of PC12 cells to NGF, further implicating the 'slow' receptor as the probable NGF binding site that elicits biological responses [59].

The ontogenesis of the plasma membrane NGF receptor has been investigated in primary cultures of neural crest cells [60,61]. Specific binding of NGF was not detected in neural crest cells at the premigratory or early migratory stage. This observation is consistent with the acquisition of differentiated neuronal functions by neural crest cells [62]. The initial appearance of NGF receptors in a subpopulation of neural crest cells after 3 to 4 days in culture was coincidental with the onset of neurotransmitter synthesis. NGF binding studies demonstrated the presence of a single receptor subtype with a binding constant similar to that of the low-affinity, 'fast' site. It has been suggested that cultured neural crest cells which have not terminally differentiated express an early progenitor form of the NGF receptor. A currently unresolved issue is whether binding of NGF to an immature receptor is sufficient by itself to promote further differentiation of the neural crest cell, or whether transformation of the primordial, low-affinity NGF receptor to the high-affinity form, considered essential for mediating the biological effects of NGF, must occur in order to produce a cellular response.

The cloning of cDNAs containing the entire coding sequence of the human membrane NGF receptor has recently been achieved [63,64]. The receptor mRNA encodes a 427 amino acid integral membrane protein with an extracellular domain, a single transmembrane domain and a cytoplasmic domain. The amino acid sequence of the extracellular domain for the human NGF receptor predicts a highly ordered structure containing a negatively charged region that may serve as the ligand-binding site. The conservation of this domain through evolution is evident and transfection of a full-length cDNA into mouse fibroblasts results in the expression of NGF receptors that are recognized by monoclonal antibodies to the human receptor and also bind NGF.

2.1.3.2.2 Nuclear receptors. Shortly after the identification of nuclear insulin receptors in insulin-responsive cells, similar observations were made in the dorsal root ganglia for NGF receptors [65]. Detailed analyses of the nuclear receptors indicated that they were of a single kinetic class and were associated with chromatin. The binding of NGF to chromatin has been recently confirmed and some characteristics of the chromatin binding site have been defined [66]. Nuclear NGF receptors have also been detected in PC12 cells [67]. Unlike dorsal root ganglion cells, the analysis of NGF binding to the PC12 nucleus depicted a more complex process. The receptors were saturable and specific and could also be subdivided into two classes on the basis of different dissociation constants. In contrast to the nuclear receptors of ganglion cells, NGF receptors found in the nuclei of PC12 cells were localized exclusively to the nuclear membrane.

The independent identification of nuclear NGF receptors on or in the nucleus has sparked a controversy regarding the meaning of these findings insofar as the putative function of nuclear NGF receptors is concerned. Several actions of NGF on target cells are transcription-mediated events and therefore involve the nucleus. It has been speculated that internalization of NGF facilitates the binding of NGF to nuclear receptors and may constitute a mechanism for initiating transcriptional events. A number of NGF-induced changes in the morphology and biochemistry of PC12 cells have been associated with structural alterations in chromatin caused by NGF. These include a decreased sensitivity of DNA to nuclease digestion and a condensation of chromatin itself [68]. While physicochemical changes in chromatin may be responsible for mediating the transcriptional events necessary to elicit the actions of NGF in target cells, most studies suggest that nearly all of the NGF internalized after binding to membrane receptors is conveyed to lysosomes and degraded [69]. The probability that a small amount of NGF could elicit a physiologically relevant signal upon reaching the nucleus cannot be excluded, however.

The potential significance of nuclear NGF receptors in PC12 cells has been inferred from experiments in which NGF was localized to the cell interior using experimental techniques that by-passed plasma membrane receptors but made NGF available for binding to nuclear sites [70,71]. The intracellular insertion of NGF, achieved by fusing NGF-responsive PC12 cells with guinea pig erythrocyte ghosts loaded with NGF or by pressure microinjection of NGF into the nucleus and cytoplasm of PC12 cells, failed to elicit the characteristic neurite out-growth. Conversely, the insertion of NGF antibody into PC12 cells, using either method, did not diminish the reactivity of these cells to extracellular NGF. Thus, NGF appears unable to initiate a biological response unless binding to plasma membrane receptors has occurred. More complex scenarios requiring second-messenger mechanisms may exist but their nature remains to be established.

2.1.3.2.3 Synaptic receptors

Persuasive though indirect evidence suggests that NGF receptors are present at the synaptic terminals of adrenergic and sensory neurons. Data supporting this concept were derived primarily from experiments on retrograde axo-plasmatic transport [72,73]. They confirmed the migration of NGF from its site of injection in areas innervated by NGF-sensitive neurons (i.e. the anterior chamber of the eye) to the cell bodies of neurons located in the ipsilateral superior cervical ganglion. The retrograde migration of NGF was consistent with the presence of functional NGF receptors at the synaptic nerve terminal.

Axo-plasmatic transport may also play a critical role in facilitating specific actions of NGF, such as the maintenance and survival of embryonic neurons and the orientation of axonal growth toward target tissues. Drugs such as 6-OHDA, guanethidine and vinblastine, all known to destroy sympathetic neurons when administered to neonatal animals, do so by preventing the retrograde transport of NGF to the neuronal cell body [74]. The neurocytotoxic effects of these agents can be antagonized by concomitant administration of NGF.

Another significant function ascribed to NGF has been its role in directing the growth of NGF-responsive axons to their target organs. A strong positive correlation has been reported between the concentrations of NGF and NGF mRNA in target organs and the density of their sympathetic innervation [75,76]. The destruction of adrenergic nerve terminals (the site of putative synaptic NGF receptors) or blockade of axonal transport by colchicine leads to a rapid increase in the NGF concentration of sympathetically innervated organs and a concomitant decrease in sympathetic ganglia [77]. It is not clear by what mechanism retrograde transport of NGF influences the direction of axonal growth. The addition of NGF to cultured neuronal cells in the vicinity of a growing neurite causes an immediate and profound alteration in the direction of axonal growth towards the source of the NGF [78]. The specific neurotrophic role of NGF in directing axonal growth has recently been complicated by studies demonstrating that NGF synthesis in developing skin, the target site of sensory neurons, was initiated only after innervation had occurred [79]. In addition, sensory neurons did not express NGF receptors until their fibres reached the cutaneous target organ. These observations appear to invalidate the hypothesis that NGF plays a primary role in directing sensory neuron axons to their target organs.

2.1.3.3 Gene regulation

The transcription of a number of genes classified as proto-oncogenes can be regulated by NGF. Proto-oncogenes contained within the normal genetic material of a cell represent genes that may be responsible for controlling signal pathways involved in the regulation of cell growth. Transformation of proto-oncogenes leads to formation of oncogenes which can alter cellular processes, so that the cell receives an inappropriate growth stimulus delivered through the normal signal pathway. Many of the products derived from oncogene transcription share sequence homology with growth factors and their receptors. The expression of two proto-oncogenes, c-myc and c-fos, is stimulated by a variety of polypeptide growth factors and other mitogenic agents. It has been suggested that the c-myc and c-fos genes were directly involved in the stimulation of mitogenesis; however, the induction of each has also been observed in the absence of cellular replication. Furthermore, c-fos expression occurs in a variety of differentiated cells that have reduced proliferative capacities.

The expression of c-fos has been selectively induced by treatment of PC12 cells with NGF [80]. Incubation of PC12 cells with NGF increased the level of c-fos mRNA within 15 min and produced a 100-fold increase 30–45 min thereafter. Pretreatment of the cells with a monoclonal antibody directed against the NGF receptor, which did not compete with NGF for binding to the receptor, blocked the induction of c-fos mRNA. This finding indicated that inhibition of the receptor-generated signal was necessary to stimulate gene transcription after NGF binding had occurred.

It is intriguing to note that microinjection of products produced by the mutated human oncogene, EJ-Ha-c-ras, into PC12 cells elicited the same response as incubation with NGF, namely neuronal differentiation and arrested growth [81]. Intracellular injections of neutralizing antibody to the gene product, $p21^{ras}$, inhibited the effects of NGF on PC12 cells [82]. The v-src oncogene also induces differentiation in this cell line. Products of the ras and src oncogenes can cause either mitogenic or differentiating responses depending upon the cell type and, in this respect, appear to resemble NGF. In certain cells, the ras oncogene product promotes growth and leads to neoplastic transformation (e.g. 3T3 cells), an effect which contrasts with that seen in PC12 cells, where it produces growth arrest and differentiation.

Based on the foregoing, it seems appropriate to conclude that the cellular responses produced by NGF are mediated via its interaction with membrane localized receptors. This process initiates a series of events that includes changes in membrane morphology, internalization of the ligand–receptor complex and possible translocation of a small portion of the receptor-bound NGF to the nucleus. The specific mechanisms responsible for transducing the signal generated by the combination of NGF with its receptor remain to be determined. Since direct introduction of free NGF into the cytoplasm and nucleus of target cells fails to elicit a biological response, presumptively, NGF must initially bind to a cell surface membrane receptor if its biological activity is to be manifest. Further, it suggests that NGF is probably not dissociated from this surface receptor following internalization of the complex. A second messenger, rather than NGF itself, probably plays a role in transduction of signals generated by the binding of NGF to its receptor site.

2.2 Exogenous factors (pharmacological agents)

An extraordinarily large number of chemical substances have been shown to influence the growth and/or differentiation of neuroblastoma cells. From a chemotherapeutic perspective, however, only those agents with high degrees of selectivity for and cytotoxic potency against neoplastic tissues warrant consideration. Consequently, a restricted group of agents with well-defined and unique biochemical mechanisms of action have been selected for discussion. These include drugs that increase cyclic nucleotide concentration (cyclic nucleotide analogues, phosphodiesterase inhibitors, prostaglandins), those that inhibit ornithine decarboxylase and hydroxymethylglutaryl coenzyme A reductase and a composite group with novel sites and mechanisms of action (merocyanine dye, phosphorylated L-dopa, desferoxamine, retinoids, purine nucleoside and dialdehyde analogues).

There is generally a tendency to consider cellular differentiation as a significant end result of any therapeutic intervention, be it initiated by growth factors or pharmacological agents. It is important to appreciate that the correlation between decreased tumorigenicity and increased cellular differentiation, as manifest by MNB neurite extrusion, for example, is not always high. Thus, agents capable of promoting the differentiation of neuroblastoma in tissue culture may not necessarily inhibit malignant expression of the tumour cell *in situ*. Pharmacologically induced increases in the intracellular cAMP levels of cultured MNB have been associated with neurite sprouting and complete loss of tumorigenicity when the cells were injected into host mice [83,84]. However, *in vitro* differentiation of MNB with dexamethasone resulted only in partial reduction of *in situ* tumorigenicity [85] and dimethylsulphoxide (DMSO), despite its potent differentiating effect on MNB, did not alter tumorigenicity [86].

2.2.1 Agents increasing cyclic AMP concentration and adenylate cyclase activity

One of the most intriguing hypotheses in tumour biology is that proposing a causal relationship between MNB cyclic AMP concentration, morphological differentiation and tumorigenicity [84]. It suggests that increases in cyclic AMP metabolism by cyclic nucleotide phosphodiesterase (PDE), resulting from increased gene expression of the latter, constitute a biochemical lesion that is associated with the malignant neuroblastoma phenotype. The experimental evidence supporting this concept was largely indirect and based primarily on the observation that dibutyryl cyclic AMP facilitated the differentiation of MNB cells [84]. Neuroblastoma cells, prior to differentiation, were found to possess extremely low levels of cyclic AMP, a phenomenon that was not due to non-responsive or uncoupled adenylate cyclase, but rather to excessive PDE hydrolytic activity [87]. Differentiation of cells correlated with an even further elevation in basal PDE activity, as well as cyclic AMP levels, a seemingly incongruous paradox. The increased cyclic AMP concentrations resulted from enhancement of cyclic AMP binding to cellular protein which served to protect the cyclic nucleotide from PDE-mediated hydrolysis.

The phosphodiesterase inhibitor 4-(-3-butoxy-4-methoxybenzyl)-2-imidazolidinone (R020-1724) induced the maturation of MNB in tissue culture and a loss of malignant potential when the cells were implanted into mice [84]. Follow-up *in situ* studies using mice inoculated with naive MNB cells (10^6/mouse) and then injected with R020-1724 around the base of the tumour have been reported [88]. This regimen increased survival (greater than 35 days) in the treated group to 60% as compared-with 10% in the control group, decreased metastases by 40% and rendered 40% of the treated mice tumour-free in contrast to none in the control group. Thus, the phosphodiesterase inhibitor (R020-174) decreased growth rate of primary MNB tumours, diminished metastatic spread and attenuated tumorigenicity *in situ*. A significant synergistic response was produced by administering prostaglandin E_1 concurrently with the PDE inhibitor. Continuous infusions of dibutyryl cyclic AMP and papaverine have been reported to suppress MNB tumour growth and enhance differentiation in recipient mice [89].

The differentiating effects produced by PGE_1 and, in particular, its inhibition of *in vitro* murine and human neuroblastoma cell growth has led to its use in some patients with Stage IV neuroblastoma [90]. A five-year-old girl with neuroblastoma was treated with papaverine, PGE_1 (50–100 ng/(kg min) i.v.) and conventional chemotherapy. This combination increased plasma cyclic AMP concentrations to a level exceeding that produced by papaverine alone. There were no data describing clinical outcome. However, the therapy was limited since the PGE_1 produced fever, nausea and abdominal pain. There have been three other reports of patients treated with long-term PGE_1 administered via intra-aortic infusion. Each subject had widespread metastatic and abdominal neuroblastoma and the PGE_1 was combined with conventional chemotherapy, making evaluation of the prostaglandin therapy difficult to ascertain. Nonetheless, both groups of investigators suggest that PGE_1 was responsible for decreasing tumour size, inducing tumour maturation and reducing the risk of tumour resection.

It is pertinent to point out deficiencies in the cyclic AMP model of MNB tumour differentiation. Many differentiating agents do not cause an increase in cyclic AMP levels [85,86]. Furthermore, some interventions that increase adenylate cyclase activity do not cause differentiation but slightly increase the rate of cell division [91]. Finally, the validity of employing high concentrations of dibutyryl cyclic AMP has been questioned. In particular, the possibility that this compound is degraded in other active substrates such as AMP and inosine or butyratel has been raised.

2.2.2 Ornithine decarboxylase inhibitors

Polyamines have long been considered to exert a significant regulatory influence on cell proliferation and possibly maturation. Derangements in polyamine metabolism brought about by agents that alter polyamine biosynthetic pathways constitute a promising approach for the development of anti-tumour agents [9]. This reasoning has led to the synthesis of ornithine decarboxylase (ODC) inhibitors because decarboxylation of l-ornithine by ODC leading to the formation of putrescine is the rate-limiting step in the biosynthesis of other polyamines, such as spermidine and spermine [93].

MNB cells induced to differentiate in tissue culture by dibutyryl cyclic AMP and the PDE inhibitor IBMX exhibit an early inhibition of putrescine uptake and a marked decrease in ODC activity and polyamine concentration [94]. It has been demonstrated that MNB cells undergo differentiation in tissue culture when incubated with a highly specific, irreversible inhibitor of ODC such as α-difluoromethylornithine [95].

Cell lines of human neuroblastoma that develop resistance to α-difluoromethylornithine also have higher rates of ODC synthesis. Recently, a human neuroblastoma cell line (Paju) has been identified that is resistant to α-difluoromethylornithine even at a concentration of 10 mM which generally inhibits the growth of all mammalian cells [96]. Since these cells had not been exposed to any other chemotherapeutic agents this report demonstrated that resistance to ODC inhibitors could occur spontaneously in neuroblastoma cell lines. Another apparent shortcoming of α-difluoromethylornithine is that it does not accumulate preferentially in tumour tissue and may inhibit polyamine biosynthesis equally well in normal and malignant tissues.

2.2.3 Dye-mediated photosensitization of MNB cells

The fluorescent dye merocyanine 540, preferentially killed MNB cells neuro2a and NB41A3 while exerting minimal toxicity on murine bone marrow cells [97]. Lethally irradiated mice reconstituted with photosensitized mixtures of MNB cells and normal bone marrow cells survived without developing tumours and were immunologically competent. The cytotoxic activity of merocyanine 540 is greater in MNB than pluripotent haemopoietic stem cells, possibly because of differences in the composition of their plasma membranes. This dye appears to bind primarily to lipid components of the membrane, exhibits little if any cell cycle specificity and is effective against cells that have become drug resistant [98].

2.2.4 Phosphorylated isomers of L-dopa

Dopa phosphates are aromatic amino acid isomers of L-dopa that contain phosphate ester linkages at positions 3 and 4 of the phenylalanine ring. These phosphorylated compounds are extremely stable and poor substrates for dopa oxidase so that they cannot be converted to melanin unless initially treated with alkaline phosphatase [99]. The cytotoxic actions of dopa phosphate derive from its conversion to L-dopa and inorganic phosphate with subsequent generation of reactive substrates during the metabolism of L-dopa to melanin.

Dopa phosphate is very effective against melanoma cells in tissue culture but extremely high concentrations (10^{-3} M) are required for its cytotoxic action. The dopa phosphates are selectively taken up into neuroectodermal cells, such as Cloudmans S91 melanoma tumour, and therefore may have therapeutic potential for other tumours such as neuroblastoma as well.

2.2.5 Mevinolin (3-hydroxy-3-methylglutaryl-coenzyme A reductase inhibitor)

The inhibition of MNB cell replication by mevinolin in tissue culture [100] and *in situ* tumours [101] has been recently reported. Administration of mevinolin (5 mg/(kg h)) by osmotic minipump significantly suppressed tumour weight to 20% of controls when compared with placebo-treated animals. The MNB tumours obtained from mevinolin-treated mice exhibited cellular degeneration and depletion of mitotic cells. The growth-inhibiting action of mevinolin appears to be unrelated to its cholesterol lowering effect since there was no change in the serum cholesterol levels of treated mice. The anti-tumour action may be due to a decrease in the synthesis of non-sterol isoprenoid compounds such as dolichol, ubiquinone, isopentenyl-tRNA or other poorly characterized isoprenoids required by rapidly proliferating cells.

2.2.6 Desferoxamine

The iron storage protein, ferritin, is frequently present in increased concentrations in the serum of patients with neuroblastoma and may constitute a useful tumour marker [102]. Ferritin is synthesized by leukaemic cells and elevations in serum levels have been demonstrated in nude mice inoculated with human neuroblastoma cells. These data suggest that ferritin is at least partially derived from neuroblastoma tumours in patients. Human neuroblastoma lines (CHP126 and CHP100), incubated with desferoxamine (60 μM) for periods of up to 5 days, had a marked decrease in cell replication rate and approximately 90% of the cells in each line were killed. The response was dose dependent and could be prevented by addition of stoichiometric amounts of ferric citrate to the medium [103]. The response of *in situ* neuroblastoma tumours to this agent has not been reported.

2.2.7 Retinoic acid and synthetic polyprenoic acid analogues

The *in vitro* induction of differentiation in human neuroblastoma cell lines has been observed following incubation with retinoic acid [104]. A new synthetic polyprenoic acid (E5166) that has properties similar to retinoic acid but is significantly less toxic has recently been investigated [105]. Retinoic acid exerts its effects presumably by interacting with nuclear DNA via binding to cellular retinoic acid binding protein. This conclusion is based on the observation that most responsive neuroblastoma cell lines, that is those which differentiate at the lowest concentration of retinoic acid, contain concentrations of cellular retinoic acid binding protein that are almost twice those observed in non-responsive neuroblastoma cell lines [106]. Other mechanisms have been proposed particularly since the report of decreased N-myc oncogene mRNA following retinoic acid induced differentiation of neuroblastoma cells [107]. Thus, it may be possible for retinoic acid to exert a direct effect on the regulation of mRNA synthesis and thereby to influence MNB cell proliferation rate and maturation [108].

The synthetic polyprenoic acid E5166 caused differentiation in two human neuroblastoma cell lines obtained from infants with stage IV disease. It is one of the most potent *in vitro* differentiating agents and is equivalent in this respect to all-*trans* retinoic acid; however, it is about 5 to 10 times less toxic than the latter.

2.2.8 Adenosine nucleoside and dialdehyde analogues

A wide variety of purine nucleoside and dialdehyde analogues have been shown to be potent inhibitors of murine neuroblastoma growth in tissue culture [108,109] and *in situ* [110]. They act primarily by inhibiting *S*-adenosylmethionine-dependent methyltransferase reactions. Significant reductions in *S*-adenosylhomocysteine hydrolase activity and increases in intracellular *S*-adenosylhomocysteine concentration have been demonstrated following incubation of neuroblastoma cells with nucleoside analogues.

The most potent nucleoside analogue investigated has been adenosine dialdehyde ($IC_{50}=1.5\times10^{-6}$ M). Dialdehydes prepared by periodic acid oxidation of their respective nucleoside have the following characteristics.

(a) The purine base from which the dialdehyde is formed determines cytotoxic activity. Thus, adenosine dialdehyde had the highest *in vitro* potency ($IC_{50}=1.5\times10^{-6}$ M) when compared with the dialdehydes of inosine, guanosine, uridine and cytidine, which had IC_{50} values ranging from 1.9×10^{-3} to 2.9×10^{-4} M.
(b) Phosphorylation of the dialdehyde did not appear to be an essential requirement from cytoxic activity since the IC_{50} values of 4′,5′-anhydro-adenosine dialdehyde and 5′-deoxyadenosine dialdehyde, which cannot undergo phosphorylation at the 5′ position, were 9.1×10^{-6} M and 7.6×10^{-6} M respectively.
(c) The presence of an active 2′,3-dialdehyde moiety appears to be essential for cytotoxic activity.

ACKNOWLEDGEMENT

This publication was partially supported by a grant from the United States Public Health Service (National Cancer Institute CA/NS44891).

REFERENCES

[1] Beckwith, J. B. & Perrin E. (1963). In situ neuroblastomas: a contribution to the natural history of neural crest tumors. *Am. J. Pathol.* **43** 1089–1104
[2] Pons, G., O'Dea, R. & Mirkin, B. L. (1982). Biological characterization of the C-1300 murine neuroblastoma: an in vivo neural crest tumor model. *Cancer Res.* **42** 3719–3723
[3] Fink, D. F. & Mirkin, B. L. (1988). Influence of host age and tumor cell burden on the growth and catecholamine content of C-1300 murine neuroblastoma in situ. *Int. J. Cancer* (in review)
[4] Schengrund, C., Repman, M. & Sheffler, B. (1979). Development of a neonatal and metastatic murine neuroblastoma model. *Cancer Res.* **39** 711–713
[5] De Potter, W. P., Fraeyman, N. H., Palm, J. W. & De Schaepdryver, A. F. (1978). Localization of noradrenaline and dopamine-β-hydroxylase in C-1300 mouse neuroblastoma. A biochemical and electron microscopic study. *Life Sci.* **23** 2665–2674
[6] Breakefield, X. O. (1976). Neurotransmitter metabolism in murine neuroblastoma cells. *Life Sci.* **18** 267–278
[7] Skaper, S. D., Adelson, G. L. & Seegmiller, J. E. (1976). Metabolism of biogenic amines in neuroblastoma and glioma cells in culture. *J. Neurochem.* **27** 1065–1070

[8] Cochard, P., Goldstein, M. & Black, I. (1979). Initial development of the noradrenergic phenotype in autonomic neuroblastoma of the rat embryo in vivo. *Devel. Biol.* **71** 100–105

[9] Pierce, G. B. (1983) The cancer cell and its control by the embryo. *Am. J. Pathol.* **113** 117–124

[10] Brinster, R. L. (1974). The effect of cells transferred into the mouse blastocyst on subsequent development. *J. Exp. Med.* **140** 1049–1056

[11] Wells, R. S. (1982). An in vitro assay of regulation of embryonal carcinoma by the blastocyst. *Cancer Res.* **42** 2736–2741

[12] Podesta, A. H., Mullins, J., Pierce, G. B. & Wells, R. S. (1984). The neurula stage mouse embryo in control of neuroblastoma. *Proc. Natl. Acad. Sci.* **81** 7608–7611

[13] Wells, R. S. & Miotto, K. A. (1986). Widespread inhibition of neuroblastoma cells in the 13 to 17-day old mouse embryo. *Cancer Res.* **46** 1659–1662

[14] Sokazaki, Y., Kato, T., Kato, H., Tanaka, R., *et al.* (1983). Characterization and partial purification of neuroblastoma growth inhibitory factor from culture medium of glioblasts. *Brain Res.* **262** 125–131

[15] Drachman, D. B. (1974). Trophic function of the neuron. *Ann N.Y. Acad Sci.* **228** 1–42

[16] Cheatle, G. L. (1903). *Br. Med. J.* **2** 1515–1516

[17] Hasson, J. (1958). The effect of methylcholanthrene on the denervated skin of strain A mice. *Cancer Res.* **18** 267–273

[18] Angeletti, P. U. & Levi-Montalcini, R. (1970). Cytolytic effect of 6-hydroxydopamine on neuroblastoma cells. *Cancer Res.* **30** 2863–2869

[19] Stein-Werblowski, R. (1974). The sympathetic nervous system and cancer. *Exp. Neurol.* **22** 97–100

[20] Batkin, S., Piette, Z. H. & Wildman, E. (1970). Effect of muscle denervation on growth of transplanted tumor in mice. *Proc. Natl. Acad Sci.* **67** 1521–1527

[21] Batkin, S. & Rayner, M. D. (1976) Mitotic changes in neuroblastoma transplanted into denervated host tissue. *Res. Comm. Chem. Path. Pharm.* **13** 145–148

[22] Chelmicka-Schorr, E. & Arnason, B. (1976). Modulatory effect of the sympathetic nervous system on neuroblastoma tumor growth. *Cancer Res.* **38** 1374–1375

[23] Fink, D. F. & Mirkin, B. L. (1987). Effects of chemical sympathectomy in neonatal and adult mice on C-1300 neuroblastoma tumor growth and catecholamine content. *Cancer Res.* **47** 5620–5625

[24] Sachs, Ch. (1973). Development of the blood–brain barrier for 6-hydroxydopamine. *J. Neurochem.* **20** 1753–1760

[25] Clark, D., Laverty, R. & Phelan, E. (1972). Long-lasting peripheral and control effects of 6-hydroxydopamine in rats. *Br. J. Pharmacol.* **44** 210–222

[26] Sachs, C. & Jonsson, G. (1975). Effects of 6-hydroxydopamine on central noradrenergic neurons during ontogeny. *Brain Res.* **99** 277–291

[27] Fink, D. F., Horn, P. & Mirkin, B. L. (1988). Differential inhibition of murine neuroblastoma tumor growth and modulation of catecholamine content following destruction of peripheral and central adrenergic neurons in neonatal mice. *J. Natl. Cancer Inst.* (in review)

[28] Chelmicka-Schorr, E., Yu, R., Sportiello, M. & Arnason, B. (1985). Sympathetic ganglia augment growth of neuroblastoma in vitro. *Europ. J. Canc. Clin. Oncol.* **21** 957–964

[29] Chelmicka-Schorr, E., Checinski, M. E., Jones, K., Yu, R. & Arnason, B. (1986). Sympathetic nervous system trophism for neuroblastoma and its age dependence in rats. *Cancer Res* **46** 5504–5506

[30] Fink, D. W. & Mirkin, B. L. (1988). Antagonism of murine neuroblastoma growth inhibition by nerve growth factor in neonatally sympathectomized mice. *Cancer Res.* (in review)

[31] Heldin, C. & Westermark, B. (1984) Growth factors: mechanism of action and relation to oncogenes. **37** 9–20

[32] Aronson, S. A. (1973). Biological characterization of mammalian cells transformed by a primate sarcoma virus. *Virology* **52** 562–567

[33] Temin, H. M. (1970). Control of multiplication of uninfected rat cells and rat cells converted by murine sarcoma virus. *J. Cell. Physiol.* **75** 107–120

[34] Cheah, M. S., Igarashi, H., Leal, F., Naharro, G. & Roberts, K. C. (1986). Growth factor-mediated proliferative pathways and the neoplastic process. *Cancer Invest.* **4** 329–341

[35] Sporn, M. B. & Roberts, A. B. (1985). Autocrine growth factors and cancer. *Nature* **313** 745–747

[36] Yankner, B. & Shooter, E. M. (1982). The biology and mechanism of action of nerve growth factor. *Ann. Rev. Biochem.* **51** 845–868

[37] Guroff, G. (1983). Nerve growth factor and other factors acting on the nervous system. In A. Lajtha (ed.) *Handbook of Neurochemistry*, vol. 5, Plenum, New York, pp. 443–466

[38] Murphy, R. A., Pantazis, N., Arnason, B. & Young, M. (1975). Secretion of a nerve growth factor by mouse neuroblastoma cells in culture. *Proc. Soc. Natl. Acad.* **72** 1895–1898

[39] Schwartz, J. P. & Costa, E. (1978). Regulation of nerve growth factor content in a neuroblastoma cell line. *Neuroscience* **3** 473–480

[40] Schwartz, J. P. (1976) Catecholamine mediated elevation of cyclic GMP in the rat CG glioma cell line. *J. Cyclic Nucl. Res.* **2** 287–296

[41] Schwartz, J. P., Chuang, D. & Costa, E. (1977). Increase in nerve growth factor content of CG glioma cells by the activation of a β-adrenergic receptor. *Brain Res.* **137** 369–375

[42] Furukawa, Y., Furukawa, S., Satoyoshi, E. & Hayashi, K. (1986). Catecholamines induce an increase in nerve growth factor content in the medium of mouse L-M cells. *J. Biol. Chem.* **261** 6039–6047

[43] Hendry, I. (1977). Cell division in the developing sympathetic nervous system. *J. Neurocytol.* **6** 299–304

[44] Levi-Montalcini, R. & Angeletti, P. U. (1968). Nerve growth factor. *Physiol. Rev.* **48** 534–569

[45] Revoltella, R. P. & Butler, R. H. (1980). Nerve growth factor may stimulate either division or differentiation of cloned C-1300 neuroblastoma cells in serum-free cultures. *J. Cell Physiol.* **104** 27–33

[46] Burstein, D. & Green, L. (1982). Nerve growth factor has both mitogenic and antimitogenic activity. *Dev. Biol.* **94** 477–482

[47] Spinelli, W., Sonnenfeld, K. H. & Ishii, D. (1982). Effects of phorbol ester tumor promoters and nerve growth factor on neurite outgrowth in cultured human neuroblastoma cells. *Cancer Res.* **42** 5067–5073

[48] Pavelic, K. & Spaventi, S. (1987) Nerve growth factor (NGF) induced differentiation of human neuroblastoma cells. *Int. J. Biochem.* **19** 1237–1240

[49] Frazier, W., Boyd, L. & Bradshaw, R. (1974). Properties of the specific binding of ^{125}I-nerve growth factor to responsive peripheral neurons. *J. Biol. Chem.* **249** 5513–5519

[50] Sutter, A. S., Riopelle, R., Harris-Warrick, R. & Shooter, E. (1979). Nerve growth factor receptors. *J. Biol.Chem.* **254** 5972–5982

[51] Block, T. & Bothwell, M. (1983). The nerve growth factor receptor on PC-12 cells: interconversion between two forms with different binding properties. *J. Neurochem.* **40** 1654–1663

[52] Bernd, P. & Green, L. A. (1984). Association of ^{125}I-nerve growth factor with PC-12 pheochromocytoma cells. *J. Biol. Chem.* **259** 15509–15516

[53] Revoltella, R., Bertolini, L., Pediconi, M. & Vigneti, E. (1974). Specific binding of nerve growth factor by murine C-1300 neuroblastoma cells. *J. Exp. Med.* **140** 437–451

[54] Sonnenfeld, K. H. & Ishii, D. S. (1985). Fast and slow nerve growth factor binding sites in human neuroblastoma and rat pheochromocytoma cell lines. Relationship of sites to each other and to neurite formation. *J. Neurosci.* **5** 1717–1728

[55] Schechter, A. L. & Bothwell, M. A. (1981). Nerve growth factor receptors on PC-12 cells: evidence for two receptor classes with differing cytoskeletal association. *Cell* **4** 867–874

[56] Landreth, G. E. & Shooter, E. M. (1980). Nerve growth factor receptors on PC-12 cells: ligand-induced conversion from low-high affinity states. *Proc. Natl. Acad. Sci. USA* **77** 4751–4755

[57] Layer, P. G. & Shooter, E. M. (1983). Binding and degradation of nerve growth factor by PC-12 pheochromocytoma cells. *J. Biol. Chem.* **258** 3012–3018

[58] Green, S. H., Rydell, R. E., Connolly, J. L. & Greene, L. A. (1986). PC-12 cell mutants that possess low — but not high affinity nerve growth factor receptors neither respond to nor internalize nerve growth factor. *J. Cell Biol.* **102** 830–843

[59] Chandler, L. P., Chandler, C. E., Hosang, M. & Shooter, E. M. (1985). A monoclonal antibody which inhibits epidermal growth factor binding has opposite effects on the biological action of epidermal growth factor in different cells. *J. Biol. Chem.* **260** 3360–3367

[60] Bernd, P. (1986). Characterization of nerve growth factor binding to cultured neural crest cells: evidence of an early developmental form of the NGF receptor. *Dev. Biol.* **115** 415–424

[61] Greiner, C. A., Lloyd, A. T. & Guroff, G. (1986). Ontogeny of the nerve growth factor receptor in primary cultures of neural crest cells. *Devlop. Brain Res.* **26** 145–150

[62] Cochard, P., Goldstein, M. & Black, I. (1979). Initial development of the noradrenergic phenotype in autonomic neuroblastomas of the rat embryo in

vivo. *Devel. Biol.* **71** 100–105
[63] Lanahan, A., Buck, C. R., Sehgal, A., Morgan, C., Mercer, E., Bothwell, M. & Chao, M. (1986). Expression and structure of the human NGF receptor. *Cell* **47** 545–554
[64] Chao, M. V., Bothwell, M. A., Ross, A. H., Koprowski, H., Lanahan, A., Buck, C. R. & Sehgal, A. (1986). Gene transfer and molecular cloning of the human NGF receptor. *Science* **232** 418–421
[65] Andres, R. Y., Jeng, I. & Bradshaw, R. (1977). NGF receptors: identification of distinct classes in plasma membranes and nuclei of embryonal dorsal root neurones. *Proc. Natl. Acad. Sci. USA* **74** 2785–2789
[66] Rakowicz-Szalczynska, E., Rodeck, U., Herlyn, M. & Koprowski, H. (1986). Chromatin binding of epidermal growth factor, nerve growth factor and platelet derived growth factor in cells bearing the appropriate surface receptor. *Proc. Natl. Acad. Sci. USA* **83** 3728–3732
[67] Yankner, B. & Shooter, E. (1979). Nerve growth factor in the nucleus: interaction with receptors on the nuclear membrane *Proc. Natl. Acad. Sci. USA* **76** 1269–1273
[68] Guroff, G., Fujita, K., Brown, I., Zabrenetsky, V., Tanner, J., Dickens, G. & Kuzuya, H. (1986). Nerve growth factor-induced nuclear changes in PC12 cells. *J. Neurosci.* (in review)
[69] Schwab, M. & Thoenen, H. (1977). Selective trans-synaptic migration of tetanus toxin after retrograde axonal transport in peripheral sympathetic nerves: a comparison with nerve growth factor. *Brain Res.* **122** 459–474
[70] Hewman, R., Schwab, M. & Thoenen, H. (1981). A second messenger required for nerve growth factor biological activity. *Nature* **292** 838–840
[71] Seeley, P., Keither, C., Shelanski, M. & Greene, L. (1983). Pressure microinjection of nerve growth factor and anti-nerve growth factor into the nucleus and cytoplasms: lack of effects on neurite outgrowth from pheochromocytomal cells. *J. Neurosci.* **3** 1488–1493
[72] Paravicin, U., Stoeckel, K. & Thoenen, H. (1975). Biological importance of retrograde axonal transport of nerve growth factor in adrenergic neurons. *Brain Res.* **84** 279–291
[73] Stoeckel, K., Guroff, G., Schwab, E. & Thoenen, H. (1976). The significance of retrograde axonal transport for the accumulation of systemically administered nerve growth factor in the rat superior cervical ganglion. *Brain Res.* **109** 271–276
[74] Johnson, E., Macia, R., Andres, R. & Bradshaw, R. (1979). The effects of drugs which destroy the sympathetic nervous system on the retrograde transport of nerve growth factor. *Brain Res.* **171** 461–472
[75] Korsching, S. & Thoenen, H. (1983). Nerve growth factor in sympathetic ganglia and corresponding target organs of the rat. Correlation with density of sympathetic innervation. *Proc. Natl. Acad. Sci. USA* **80** 3515–3516
[76] Shelton, D. & Reichardt, L. (1984). Expression of the β-adrenergic nerve growth factor gene correlates with the density of sympathetic innervation in effector organs. *Proc. Natl. Acad. Sci. USA* **81** 7951–7955
[77] Korsching, S. & Thoenen, H. (1985). Treatment with 6-hydroxydopamine and colchicine decreases nerve growth factor levels in sympathetic ganglia and

increases them in the corresponding target tissues. *J. Neurosci.* **5** 1058–1061
[78] Letourneau, P. (1978). Chemotactic response of nerve fiber elongation to nerve growth factor. *Develop. Biol.* **66** 183–196
[79] Davies, A. M., Bandtlow, C., Heumann, R., Korsching, S., Rohrer, H. & Thoenen, H. (1987). Timing and site of nerve growth factor synthesis in developing skin in relation to innervation and expression of the receptor. *Nature* **326** 353–358
[80] Curran, T. & Morgan, G. (1985). Superinduction of C-fos by nerve growth factor in the presence of peripherally active benzodiazepines. *Science* **229** 1265–1268
[81] Bar-Sagi, D. & Feramisco, J. R. (1985). *Cell* **42** 841
[82] Hagag, N., Halegoua, S. & Viola, H. (1986). Inhibition of growth factor induced differentiation of PC12 cells by microinjection of antibody to ras p21. *Nature* **319** 680–682
[83] Prasad, K. N. (1972). Cyclic-AMP induced differentiated mouse neuroblastoma cells lose tumorigenic characteristics. *Cytobios* **6** 163–166
[84] Prasad, K. N., Sahu, S. K. & Sinha, P. K. (1976). Cyclic nucleotides in the regulation of expression of differentiated functions in neuroblastoma. *J. Natl. Cancer Inst.* **57** 619–629
[85] Sandquist, D. & Black, A. C. (1982). Reduced tumorigenicity of cultured neuroblastoma cells after treatment in vitro with dexamethasone. *Fed. Proc.* **41** 1107–1114
[86] Danon, Y. L. & Kaminsky, E. (1985). Dimethyl sulfoxide-induced differentiation does not alter tumorigenicity of neuroblastoma cells. *J. Neuro-Oncology* **3** 43–51
[87] Prasad, K. N. (1975). Differentiation of neuroblastoma cells in culture. *Biol. Rev.* **50** 129–265
[88] Anderson, D. W. & Crowle, A. J. (1982). Regression and differentiation of neuroblastoma tumors in mice treated with differentiating agents — prostaglandin E_1 and a phosphodiesterase inhibitor. *Cancer Lett.* **16** 287–295
[89] Nakajima, F., Imashuku, S., Webber, B. & Green, A. A. (1982). In vivo effect of continuous infusion of Bt_2 cAMP-papaverine on growth and differentiation of C-1300 neuroblastoma. *Proc. Am. Assn. Cancer Res.* **23** 37
[90] Imashukuk, S., Todo, S., Esumi, N., Hashida, T., Tsunamoto, K. & Nakajima, F. (1985). Tumor differentiation — application of prostaglandins in the treatment of neuroblastoma. In: A. Evans, G. D'Angio & R. Seeger (eds.) *Advances in Neuroblastoma Research*, Alan R. Liss, New York, pp. 89–99
[91] Murphy, N. G. (1986). Studies of the regulation of basal adenylate cyclase activity by membrane polyunsaturated fatty acids in cultured neuroblastoma. *J. Neurochem.* **47** 245–253
[92] Pegg, A. E. (1988). Polyamine metabolism and its importance in neoplastic growth and as a target for chemotherapy. *Cancer Res.* **48** 759–775
[93] Porter, C. W. & Supfrin, J. R. (1986). Interference with polyamine synthesis and/or function by analogs of polyamines or methionine as a potential anticancer chemotherapeutic strategy. *Anticancer Res.* **6** 525–542
[94] Chen, K. Y. & Rinehart, C. A., (1981). Difference in putrescine transport in undifferentiated versus differentiated mouse NB-15 neuroblastoma cells.

Biochem. Biophys. Res. Commun. **101** 243–249
[95] Chen, K. Y., Nau, D. & Liu, A. (1983). Effects of inhibitors of ornithine decarboxylase on the differentiation of mouse neuroblastoma cells. *Cancer Res.* **43** 2812–2818
[96] Poso, H., Karvonen, E., Suomalainen, H. & Andersson, L. (1984). A human neuroblastoma cell line with altered ornithine decarboxylase. *J. Biol. Chem.* **259** 12307–12310
[97] Sieber, F. & Sieber-Blum, M. (1986). Dye-mediated photosensitization of murine neuroblastoma cells. *Cancer Res.* **46** 2072–2076
[98] Valinsky, J. E., Easton, T. G. & Reich, E. (1978). Merocyanine 540 as a fluorescent probe of membranes: selective staining of leukemic and immature hemopoietic cells. *Cell* **13** 487–500
]99] Pawelek, J. M. & Murray, M. (1986). Increase in melanin formation and promotion of cytotoxicity in cultured melanoma cells caused by the phophorylated isomers of L-dopa. *Cancer Res.* **46** 493–497
[100] Maltese, W. A. (1984). Induction of differentiation in murine neuroblastoma cells by melvinolin, a competitive inhibitor of 3-hydroxy-3-methylglutaryl-coenzyme A reductase. *Biochem. Biophys. Res. Commun.* **120** 454–460
[101] Maltese, W. A., Defendi, R., Green, R. A., Sheridan, K. M. & Donley, D. K. (1985). Suppression of murine neuroblastoma growth in vivo by merinolin, a competitive inhibitor of 3-hydroxy-3-methylglutaryl-coenzyme A reductase. *J. Clin. Invest.* **76** 1748–1754
[102] Hann, H., Stahlhut, V. A. & Evans, A. E. (1985) Serum ferritin as a prognostic indicator in neuroblastoma: biological effects of isoferritins. In: A. E. Evans, G., D'Angio & R. C. Seeger (eds.) *Advances in Neuroblastoma Research*, Alan R. Liss, New York, pp. 331–345
[103] Blatt, J. & Stitely, S. (1987). Antineuroblastoma activity of desferoxamine in human cell lines. *Cancer Res.* **47** 1749–1750
[104] Sidell, N. (1981). Retinoic acid induced growth inhibition and morphologic differentiation of human neuroblastoma cells in vitro. *J. Natl. Cancer Inst.* **68** 589–596
[105] Sugimoto, T., Sawada, T., Matsumura, T., Horii, Y., Kemshead, J. T., Suzuki, Y., Okada, M., Tagaya, O. & Hino, T. (1987). Morphological differentiation of human neuroblastoma cell lines by a new synthetic polyprenoic acid (E5166). *Cancer Res.* **47** 5433–5438
[106] Sidell, N., Lucas, C. A. & Kreutzberg, G. W. (1984). Regulation of acetylcholinesterase activity by retinoic acid in a human neuroblastoma cell line. *Exp. Cell Res.* **155** 305–309
[107] Thiele, C. J., Reynolds, C. P. & Israel, M. A. (1985). Decreased expression of N-myc precedes retinoic acid-induced morphological differentiation of human neuroblastoma. *Nature* **313** 404–406
[108] O'Dea, R. F., Mirkin, B. L., Hogenkamp, H. P. & Barten, D. M. (1987). Effect of adenosine analogues on protein carboxylmethyltransferase, S-adenosylhomocysteine hydrolase and ribonucleotide reductase activity in murine neuroblastoma cells. *Cancer Res.* **47** 3656–3661
[109] Mirkin, B. L., O'Dea, R. F. & Hogenkamp, H. P. (1987). Cytotoxic action of adenosine nucleoside and dialdehyde analogues on murine neuroblastoma in

tissue culture: structure–action relationships. *Cancer Res.* **47** 3650–3655
[110] Bostrom, B. C., Hogenkamp, H. P. & Mirkin, B. L. (1988). Inhibitory effect of adenosine dialdehyde on in situ murine neuroblastoma growth. *Cancer Res.* (in review)

7

Depletion of neuroblastoma cells from bone marrow aspirates by physical cell separation and immunorosetting

Carl G. Figdor*, Ineke C. M. Slaper-Cortenbach† and Ria Wijngaarden-DuBois†
* The Netherlands Cancer Institute, Antoni van Leeuwenhoek Huis, Plesmanlaan 121, 1066 CX Amsterdam, The Netherlands; and
† Central Laboratory of The Netherlands Red Cross Blood Transfusion Service, Plesmanlaan 125, 1066 CX Amsterdam, The Netherlands

1. INTRODUCTION

Treatment of cancer patients with potentially curative high doses of chemotherapy is often accompanied by unacceptable high toxicity to normal tissues such as the bone marrow compartment, which plays an essential role in haematopoiesis. To overcome this specific problem the haematopoietic precursor cells can be rescued by aspiration of bone marrow prior to treatment and by re-infusion after therapy. This so-called autologous bone marrow transplantation has already been applied in combination with high dose chemotherapy to treat patients with solid malignancies [1–3]. However, for tumours that tend to spread to the bone marrow compartment, or for haematological disorders, the value of this kind of treatment is limited [4]. In these cases this treatment modality is only applicable to those patients with a completely disease-free bone marrow. Therefore during the past five years much effort has been spent on the development of methods to clean contaminated bone marrow *in vitro*, which will undoubtedly lead to a more general use of autologous bone marrow transplantation in combination with high dose chemotherapy.

Various methods have been developed to kill or remove tumour cells that contaminate bone marrow suspensions. In principle three different ways are open for the manipulation of autologous bone marrow *in vitro*: pharmacological, immunological and physical methods. One of the advantages of bone marrow manipulation *in vitro* is also that pharmaceuticals which are less well tolerated *in vivo* can be applied. However, until now most investigators have attempted to use monoclonal antibodies for *in vitro* bone marrow cleaning. Monoclonal antibodies have been used in different ways. First, tumour cells can be removed by complement-mediated lysis [5,6]. Secondly, monoclonal antibodies have been conjugated to toxins or to chemotherapeutic compounds in order to eliminate tumour cells [7,8]. More recently, malignant cells were coated with anti-tumour antibodies and indirectly formed rosettes with cobalt- or iron-containing beads coated with anti-mouse antibodies. These rosettes can be removed from the bone marrow suspensions by means of strong magnets [9–11].

Furthermore, differences in the physical properties between tumour cells and bone marrow stem cells (cell size and cell density) can be exploited to clear the bone marrow of contaminating tumour cells [12]. Recently immunological and physical methods were combined by applying tetramolecular complexes of monoclonal antibodies to form rosettes of tumour cells with human red blood cells [13]. Subsequently, the rosetted tumour cells were removed by density gradient centrifugation.

Although impressive results have been obtained in cleaning up contaminated bone marrow, we feel that none of the methods mentioned above will be efficacious enough on its own to remove virtually all solid tumour cells in bone marrow aspirates. For example, it was shown by Buckman *et al.* [14] that small clumps of tumour cells (micrometastases) were not efficiently eliminated by monoclonal antibodies conjugated to a toxin, probably because of a less effective penetration of the conjugate. However, if a physical cell separation technique had been applied in advance, aggregates of cells would have been removed. Therefore we propose to combine two or more methods to eliminate tumour cells, preferably methods exploiting different properties of the tumour cells. In the present study we apply a powerful physical cell separation technique, centrifugal elutriation, which allows processing of large numbers of bone marrow cells. This step results in a complete removal of all tumour cell aggregates and in addition removes the majority of the tumour cells from the bone marrow stem cells. Subsequently we applied tetramolecular complexes of monoclonal antibodies to eliminate the remaining tumour cells by the formation of rosettes which were separated from the concentrated bone marrow progenitor cells.

2. RESULTS AND DISCUSSION

2.1 Concentration of bone marrow progenitor cells by centrifugal elutriation

It is evident that, no matter which cleaning procedure is used, good results can only be achieved if the bone marrow suspension is optimally prepared. In the first place this requires the removal of red blood cells which constitute the largest number of cells and which are not required for successful engraftment. Furthermore, an attempt should be made to concentrate the bone marrow progenitor cells in a small volume to facilitate further *in vitro* manipulation. To remove the red blood cells from the bone marrow aspirates, we applied a blood component separator to prepare a buffy coat from the bone marrow suspension. As described previously this resulted in a >95% removal of the red blood cells, whereas >90% of the stem cells remained in the buffy coat [12,15]. Alternatively, the bone marrow aspirates were centrifuged over a Ficoll–Hypaque mixture to prepare a mononuclear cell suspension. Thus concentrated cell suspensions were loaded into an elutriator rotor [16] to purify further the haematopoietic progenitor cells. Results of a representative experiment are shown in Table 1. In general six fractions were obtained. The majority of the

Table 1 — Distribution of fractionated fresh or frozen mononuclear cells obtained from bone marrow suspensions separated by centrifugal elutriation

Fraction	RPM	Fresh bone marrow		Frozen bone marrow	
		% WBC	% CFU-c	% WBC	% CFU-c
1	2900	31	—	25	—
2	2650	20	<1	12	<1
3	2400	9	73	14	48
4	2150	8	12	12	35
5	1900	8	8	11	12
6	0	24	6	26	4

Separation was carried out at 10°C and at a constant flow rate of 18 ml/min by intermittently (10 min intervals) decreasing the rotor speed [16,17]. The number of white blood cells (WBC) was determined by electronic sizing (Coulter counter) and the number of progenitor cells was obtained by determination of the number of myeloid progenitor cells (CFU-c) after ten days of culture [15]. The values represent the percentage of the recovered cells.

progenitor cells were obtained in fraction 3 and a small but significant number of CFU-c were obtained in fraction 4. Together these fractions generally contained 70–90% of the CFU-c, which became four- to five-fold concentrated since fractions 3 and 4 constituted only 20–25% of the initial number of nucleated cells. In addition we tested whether centrifugal elutriation was also suited to concentrate CFU-c from already-frozen mononuclear cell suspensions derived from marrow harvested from neuroblastoma patients. The data in Table 1 show that identical results were obtained with the exception of the observed tendency of frozen marrow to form loose cell aggregates, resulting in a somewhat lower yield.

2.2 Bone marrow cleaning by means of centrifugal elutriation

To study whether centrifugal elutriation was suitable not only to concentrate bone marrow progenitor cells but also to remove tumour cells from contaminated marrow, we mixed bone marrow cells with neuroblastoma cells. The result of this separation is illustrated in Fig. 1, where the size distributions of the bone marrow cells, the tumour cells and the fractionated cells are shown. Table 2 shows the results of an experiment in which a mixture of 90% bone marrow cells and 10% cultured neuroblastoma cell line cells (CHP-212) was separated. It becomes clear from Table 2 that the CFU-c were concentrated in fractions 3 and 4, but that these fractions contained only 11% of the contaminating neuroblastoma cells. Furthermore, we observed that fraction 6 contained small aggregates of tumour cells, whereas fractions 3 and 4 were virtually

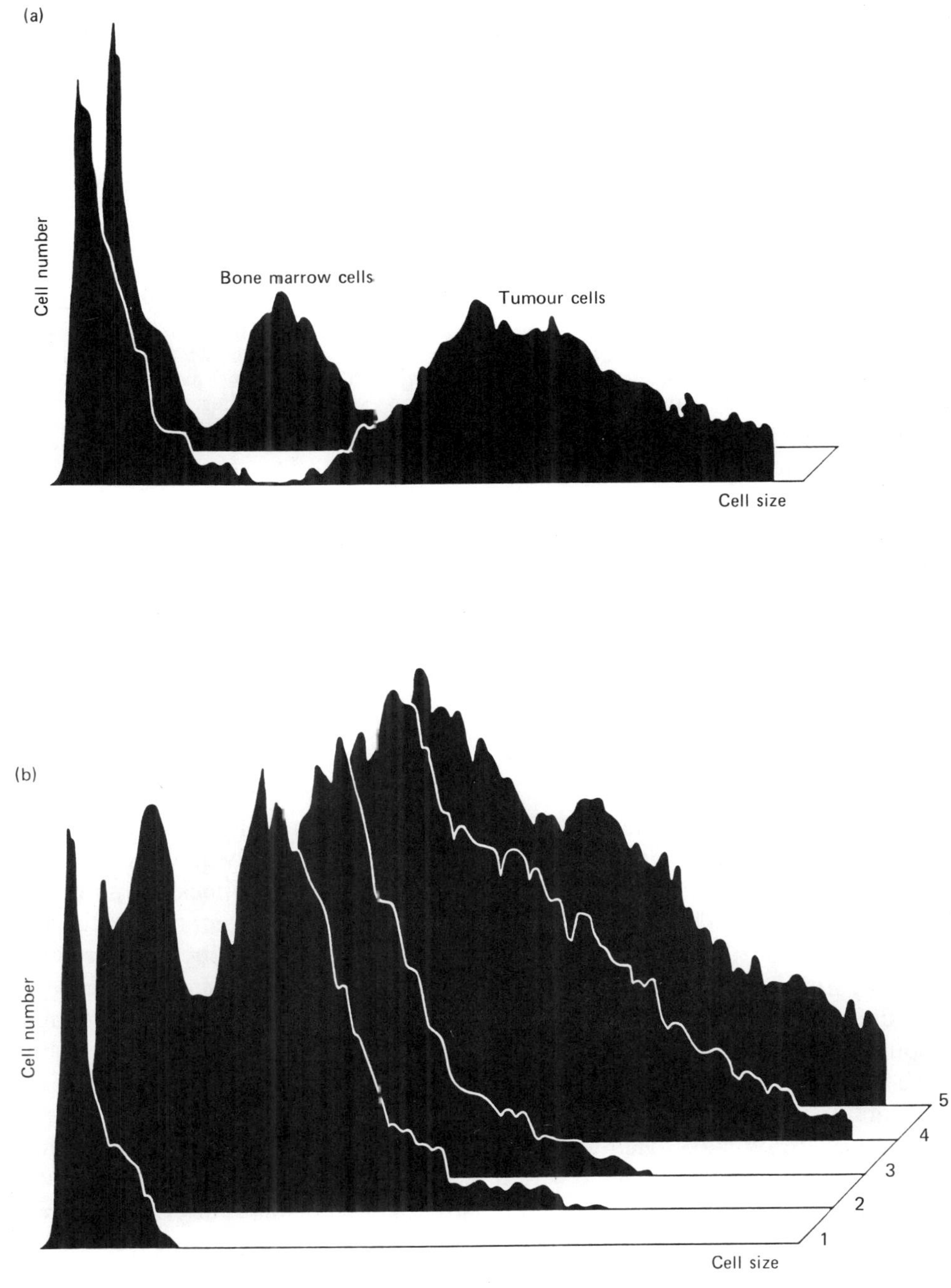

Fig. 1 — Size distribution of (a) mononuclear bone marrow cells and CHP-212 neuroblastoma cells and (b) fractionated bone marrow (five fractions are shown) which contain 10% CHP-212 cells. The size distribution was measured by Coulter counter and channelyser.

Table 2 — The distribution of CFU-c and neuroblastoma cells after fractionation by centrifugal elutriation

Fraction	RPM	% CFU-c	% CHP-212 cells
1	2900	<1	<1
2	2650	5	<1
3	2400	67	2
4	2150	12	9
5	1900	6	45
6	0	9	42

Mononuclear cells derived from bone marrow were mixed in a 10:1 ratio with cultured neuroblastoma cells (CHP-212). 150×10^6 cells were separated by centrifugal elutriation. The number of CFU-c was determined by indirect immunofluorescence after staining with a monoclonal antibody (NKI-neu1) specifically reacting with neuroblastoma cells in combination with FITC-conjugated goat anti-mouse antibodies ($F(ab)_2$ fragments). The data represent the percentage of the recovered CFU-c and neuroblastoma cells.

devoid of cell aggregates. These results justify the conclusion that centrifugal elutriation is suited to remove the greater part of tumour cells from contaminated bone marrow suspensions and eliminates all cell aggregates. However, additional methods are required to remove the remaining tumour cells from this single-cell bone marrow suspension.

2.3 Monoclonal antibodies directed against neuroblastoma-associated antigens

To purify further the concentrated bone marrow suspension we have chosen to exploit differences in the expression of cell surface antigens between bone marrow stem cells and neuroblastoma cells. To this end mice were repeatedly immunized with neuroblastoma cell line cells (CHP-212). Subsequently, hybridomas secreting monoclonal antibodies were prepared according to a previously described protocol [18]. The hybridomas were selected for the secretion of monoclonal antibodies reacting with neuroblastoma cells but not with normal bone marrow cells. Five hybridomas were obtained termed NKI-neu1-5 (see Table 3). Antibodies secreted by these hybridomas stained (immunofluorescence) neuroblastoma cells (CHP-212) and did not react with normal blood and bone marrow cells, except for a minor population (<1%) of as-yet unidentified bone marrow cells. Further examination revealed that three of the five hybridomas secreted antibodies that were highly specific for neuroblastoma and other neuroectodermal tissues, and that all three antibodies are directed against the same cell surface antigen [manuscript in preparation]. The antibodies reacted with frozen tissue sections of neuroblastoma cells and showed some reactivity with other tumours of neuroectodermal origin (Table 3). The antibodies neu4 and neu5 seemed less specific since they cross-reacted with various normal tissues. Finally, it was demonstrated that the antibodies did not inhibit the growth of CFU-c (not shown).

2.4 Bone marrow cleaning by immunorosetting

The monoclonal antibodies described above were used to remove specifically neuroblastoma cells from bone marrow aspirates. Recently impressive results have

Table 3 — Reaction pattern of five anti-neuroblastoma antibodies (NKI-neu1-5)

Cell type	Reactivity with				
	neu1	neu2	neu3	neu4	neu5
White blood cells	–	–	–	–	–
Red blood cells	–	–	–	–	–
Thrombocytes	–	–	–	–	–
Bone marrow cells[a]	–	–	–	–	–
Cell lines					
Neuroblastoma	+	+	+	+	+
Melanoma[b]	+/–	+/–	+/–	+/–	+/–
B cell lines	–	–	–	–	+/–
Tissue sections					
Neuroblastoma	+	+	+	+	+
Normal tissue	–[c]	–[c]	–[c]	+[d]	+[d]

The specificity of the antibodies was determined by means of indirect immunofluorescence (cell lines) and by peroxidase staining (tissue sections).

[a] Occasionally a small number (<1%) of the bone marrow cells stained positively with neu1-5.
[b] Four out of six melanoma cell lines stained positive with neu1-4, and five out of six cell lines with neu5.
[c] Neul-3 showed reactivity with only normal brain and nerve tissue.
[d] Neu4 and neu5 reacted with a variety of tissues including nerve, brain, kidney and connective tissue.

been obtained with cobalt- or iron-containing beads coated with anti-mouse immunoglobulins. Here we apply a different immunorosetting technique. Instead of iron-containing beads, human erythrocytes were used to form rosettes. Therefore two monoclonal antibodies of the IgG1 subclass (one directed against glycophorin A of the human erythrocyte, the other directed against neuroblastoma) were cross-linked by a rat anti-mouse IgG1 monoclonal antibody, resulting in the formation of a tetramolecular complex [13]. These complexes were loaded on human erythrocytes and after addition of neuroblastoma cells, immune rosettes were formed. The formed rosettes are strong enough to withstand the centrifugal forces that occur during density gradient centrifugation and can be removed effectively from the normal haematopoietic progenitor cells. Until now this method has successfully been applied to remove leukaemic tumour cells from bone marrow by using anti-cALLA (CD10) and anti-pan B (CD19) antibodies [19, manuscript in preparation].

Table 4 shows the results of experiments in which CHP-212 neuroblastoma cells were added to mononuclear bone marrow cells. The data in Table 4 demonstrate that, although some depletion of CHP-212 cells is observed, more than 50% of the contaminating tumour cells remained in the cell suspension, which indicates that the rosette technique was unable to eliminate the tumour cells efficiently. This is in contrast with the results obtained after purging of marrow mixed with non-adherent cALLA positive cell line cells [19]. From these results it was concluded that immunorosetting was less suitable to remove neuroblastoma cells than leukaemic

Table 4 — The effect of immunorosette depletion on a mixture of normal bone marrow cells and CHP-212 cells

Treatment	% CHP-212 cells
(1) Erythrocytes + neu1	12
(2) Erythrocytes + neu2	17
(3) Erythrocytes + neu1 + neu2	14
(4) Uncoated erythrocytes	25

Immunorosetting was carried out using NKI-neu1 or NKI-neu2 antibodies, or both. The number of remaining CHP-212 cells was determined by immunofluorescence. Uncoated erythrocytes were used as control.

cells. The most likely explanation is the tendency of neuroblastoma cells to form cell aggregates with other neuroblastoma cells or with bone marrow cells. Apparently the number of erythrocytes bound to these cell aggregates is too low to allow efficient separation.

2.5 Bone marrow cleaning by centrifugal elutriation and immunorosetting

Finally, we carried out an experiment in which both techniques were sequentially applied. We used defrosted mononuclear bone marrow cells of a neuroblastoma patient. These bone marrow cells were free of tumour cells as judged by immunofluorescence after labelling with anti-neuroblastoma antibodies. Therefore cultured CHP-212 cells were added.

The following experiment was conducted. Part of the cell suspension was subjected to immunorosetting in order to investigate the efficacy of this method. The remainder of the cell suspension was separated by centrifugal elutriation to concentrate the bone marrow progenitor cells and to remove cell aggregates and part of the tumour cells. Subsequently fractions 2–4, which contained the majority of the bone marrow stem cells, were subjected to immunorosetting. The data shown in Table 5 demonstrate that immunorosetting alone cannot adequately remove the neuroblastoma cell from the bone marrow suspension and confirm the results of the experiments listed in Table 4. Fraction 3 which contained 42.8% of the CFU-c is almost free of tumour cells. Fraction 4, however, which constituted 31.9% of the CFU-c, still contained a considerable number of neuroblastoma cells. However, if we first apply centrifugal elutriation to remove cell aggregates, the remaining tumour cells are sensitive to elimination by immunorosetting. The results in Table 5 show that these tumour cells can be eliminated by the immunorosetting technique, resulting in a bone marrow suspension that contains less than 0.5×10^3 clonogenic units/10^6 cells, in comparison with the 0.5×10^5 clonogenic units/10^6 cells of the original bone marrow suspension. These results demonstrate the potency of a multimodal approach. Immunorosetting, which in itself seems ineffective in removing neuroblastoma cells, can be applied for purging procedures of solid tumours provided that the cell suspension is free of aggregates, which, in our case, was accomplished by centrifugal elutriation.

Table 5 — Depletion of CHP-212 cells from bone marrow by centrifugal elutriation and immunorosetting

Fractions	CFU-GM[a] %	CHP-212[b]	
CE fraction 1	—	7	
2	1	12	
3	42.8	14	
4	31.9	7.8×10^4	
5	17.9	1.1×10^5	
6	6.4	2.9×10^6	
Mixed cell suspension: 10^6 cells[c]	100	0.3×10^5[d]	
Ficoll[e]	80	0.8×10^5[d]	
Ficoll CE fractions 2–3	ND[f]	24[d]	0.5×10^3
Ficoll CE fraction 4	ND	480[d]	

A mixture of bone marrow cells and CHP-212 cells was separated by centrifugal elutriation (CE) into six fractions. Subsequently, fractions 2 + 3 and 4 were subjected to immunorosetting and separated over Ficoll ($d = 1.077$).

[a] CFU-GM: total of clusters (>20 cells) and colonies (>40 cells).
[b] CHP-212: recovery of clonogenic units after elutriation and/or immunorosette depletion [6].
[c] Untreated cell suspension.
[d] Clonogenic units per 10^6 plated cells.
[e] Cells subjected to immunorosetting alone.
[f] ND: not determined.

3. CONCLUDING PERSPECTIVES

It has already been shown by Buckman *et al.* [14] that single-cell suspensions are a prerequisite to exploit optimally the capacity of monoclonal antibodies to deplete bone marrow of contaminating tumour cells. Here we show that immunorosetting, a technique well suited to remove leukaemic cells from bone marrow aspirates, is ineffective in eliminating neuroblastoma cells. However, if this method is preceded by centrifugal elutriation, in order to prepare a single-cell suspension, the remaining tumour cells can be removed by immunorosetting. This illustrates the advantage of a multimodal approach in which different methods, each exploiting distinct properties of tumour cells (i.e. cell surface antigens, cell size, cell density, sensitivity to pharmaceuticals) are combined to achieve a maximum result.

It is obvious that, provided that no progenitor cells are lost, a reduction of the number of cells in the bone marrow aspirate increases the efficacy of other methods to remove specifically contaminating tumour cells. In addition, the less manipulation is needed, the more methods can be applied without affecting the viability of the stem cells and their capacity to reconstitute the bone marrow compartment. A simple way of reducing the cell number is exploiting the differences in cell density by preparing a buffy coat of the bone marrow aspirate. We showed previously that it is possible to reduce the number of erythrocytes by 95% without losing more than 10% of the haematopoietic progenitor cells by using a blood component separator to prepare a buffy coat [12,15]. The results of the present study demonstrate that further separation of thus-prepared bone marrow suspensions by centrifugal elutriation, which separates cells mainly according to cell size, leads to five-fold concentration of the progenitor cells. It can be calculated that, if both techniques are applied, a 10–20-fold concentration of the bone marrow progenitor cells is obtained with respect to the number of red blood cells. The advantages of both methods are that they can process large numbers of cells and can be carried out without using body-foreign substances and with minimal manipulation of the bone marrow cells. Furthermore, we demonstrated that centrifugal elutriation not only is extremely well suited to concentrate the haematopoietic precursor cells but also removes the majority of contaminating neuroblastoma cells and, more importantly, removes all cell aggregates, thus facilitating further bone marrow clearing by immunological methods such as immunorosetting. Current studies are aimed at adapting both methods for clinical application. In our opinion, the concentration of haematopoietic precursor cells by physical cell separations, such as those described above, should precede any other method to remove specifically solid tumour cells from autologous bone marrow suspensions to obtain optimal results.

ACKNOWLEDGEMENTS

We thank Martin de Boer, Karin Ham, Jane Kerr, Richard Reijneke and Ferry Bergkamp for technical assistance and Marie Anne van Halem for secretarial help.

This work was supported by a grant from the 'Koningin Wilhelmina Fonds' (The Netherlands Cancer Foundation), Grant NKI 84-5, and by the SKK Foundation for Pediatric Cancer Research.

Dr. J. de Kraker from the Emma Kinder Ziekenhuis, Amsterdam, is acknowledged for the neuroblastoma specimens.

REFERENCES

[1] Spitzer, G., Dicke, K. A., Litam, J., Verma, D. S., Zander, A., Lanzotti, V., Valdivieso, M., McCredie, K. B. & Samules, M. L. (1980). High-dose combination chemotherapy with autologous bone marrow transplantation in adult solid tumors. *Cancer* **45** 3075

[2] Souhami, R. L., Harper, P. G., Linch, D., Trask, C., Goldtone, A. H., Tobias, J., Spiro, S. G., Geddes, D. M. & Richards, J. D. M. (1982). High dose cyclophosphamide with autologous marrow transplantation as initial treatment of small cell carcinoma of the bronchus. *Cancer Chemother. Pharmacol.* **8** 31

[3] Glode, L. M., Robinson, W. A., Hartmann, D. W., Klein, J. J., Thomas, M. R. & Morton, N. (1982). Autologous bone marrow transplantation in the therapy of small cell carcinoma of the lung. *Cancer Res.* **42** 4270

[4] Pritchard, J., McElwain, T. J. & Graham-Pole, J. (1982). High-dose melphalan with autologous marrow for treatment of advanced neuroblastoma. *Br. J. Cancer* **46** 86

[5] Ritz, J., Bast, R. C., Clavell, L. A., Hercend, T., Sallen, S. E., Lipton, J. M., Feeney, M., Nathan, D. G. & Schlossman, S. F. (1982) Autologous bone marrow transplantation in CALLA-positive acute lymphoblastic leukaemia

after in-vitro treatment with J5 monoclonal antibody and complement. *Lancet* **2** 60–63

[6] Bast, R. C., Jr., De Fabritiis, P., Lipton, J., Gelber, R., Maver, C., Nadler, L., Sallen, S. & Ritz, J. (1985). Elimination of malignant clonogenic cells from human bone marrow using multiple monoclonal antibodies and complement. *Cancer Res.* **45** 499–503

[7] Embleton, M. J., Rowland, G. F., Simmonds, R. G., Jacobs, E., Marsden, C. H. & Baldwin, R. W. (1983). Selective cytotoxicity against human tumour cells by a vindesine-monoclonal antibody conjugate. *Br. J. Cancer* **47** 943

[8] Yeager, A. M., Wiley, J. M., Jones, R., Rowley, S. D., Zuehlsdorf, M., Colvin, O. M. & Santos, G. W. (1987). Pharmacologic treatment of bone marrow to eliminate clonogenic tumor cells: laboratory and clinical studies. In: A. P. Gee & S. Gross (eds.) *Bone Marrow Transplantation,* vol. 2, suppl. 2, Macmillan, Basingstoke, pp. 34–38

[9] Poynton, C. H., Dicke, K. A., Culbert, S., Frankel, L. S., Jagannath, S. & Reading, C. L. (1983). Immunomagnetic removal of CALLA positive cells from human bone marrow. *Lancet* **1** 524

[10] Treleaven, J. G., Ugelstad, J., Philip, T., Gibson, F. M., Rembaum, A., Caine, G. D. & Kemshead, J. T. (1984). Removal of neuroblastoma cells from bone marrow with monoclonal antibodies conjugated to magnetic microspheres. *Lancet* **1** 70–73

[11] Kemshead, J. T., Heath, L., Gibson, F. M., Katz, F., Richmond, F., Treleaven, J. G. & Ugelstad, J. (1986). Magnetic microspheres and monoclonal antibodies for the depeletion of neuroblastoma cells from bone marrow. Experience, improvements and observations. *Br. J. Cancer* **54** 771–778

[12] Figdor, C. G., Voûte, P. A., De Kraker, J., Vernie, L. N. & Bont, W. S. (1985). Physical cell separation of neuroblastoma cells from bone marrow. In: *Advances in Neuroblastoma Research*, Alan R. Liss, New York, pp. 459–470

[13] Lansdorp, P. M., Aalberse, R. C., Bos, R., Schutter, W. & Van Bruggen, E. F. J. (1986). Cyclic tetramolecular complexes of monoclonal antibodies, a new type of cross-linking reagent. *Eur. J. Immunol.* **16** 679–683

[14] Buckman, R., Shepherd, V., Coombes, R. C., McIlhinney, R. A. J., Patel, S. & Neville, A. M. (1982). Elimination of carcinoma cells from human bone marrow. *Lancet* **2** 1428–1430

[15] Figdor, C. G., De Witte, T., Raymakers, R., Haanen, C. & Bont, W. S. (1985). Concentration of hematopoietic progenitor cells from human bone marrow by a new type of blood component separator. *Vox Sang.* **49** 154–160

[16] Figdor, C. G., Bont, W. S., De Vries, J. E. & Van Es, W. L. (1981). Isolation of large numbers of highly purified lymphocytes and monocytes with a modified centrifugal elutriation technique. *J. Immunol. Methods* **40** 275–288

[17] Figdor, C. G., Van Es, W. L., Leemans, J. M. M. & Bont, W. S. (1984). A centrifugal elutriation system of separating small numbers of cells *J. Immunol. Methods* **68** 73–87

[18] Keizer, G. D., Borst, J., Figdor, C. G., Spits, H., Miedema, F., Terhorst, C. & De Vries, J. E. (1985). Biochemical and functional characteristics of the human leukocyte membrane antigen family LFA-1, Mo-1 and p150,95. *Eur. J. Immunol.* **15** 1142–1147

[19] Slaper-Cortenbach, I. C. M., Admiraal, L. G., Von dem Borne, A. E. G. Kr., Van Leeuwen, E. F., Engelfriet, C. P. & Tetteroo, P. A. T. (1987). A new immunorosette technique for the depletion of leukemic cells from autologous bone marrow grafts. In: A. P. Gee & S. Gross (eds.) *Bone Marrow Transplantation*, vol. 2, suppl. 2, Macmillan, Basingstoke, p. 141

8

Radionuclide treatment of neuroblastoma using [^{131}I]*meta*-iodobenzylguanidine

C. A. Hoefnagel, J. de Kraker and **P. A. Voûte,**
Department of Nuclear Medicine and Werkgroep Kindertumoren, The Netherlands Cancer Institute, 1066 CX Amsterdam, The Netherlands

1. INTRODUCTION

Meta-iodobenzylguanidine (MIBG), a guanethidine analogue, labelled with iodine-131 [^{131}I], has been successfully used for the diagnosis and treatment of phaeochromocytoma [1, 2]. This led to its use in other tumours which are derived from the neural crest and are capable of concentrating this radiopharmaceutical in the neurosecretory granules.

From the embryonic development it can be concluded that tumours arising from the neural crest may be located throughout the body and present as many different clinical syndromes. Table 1 gives a list of neural crest tumours. Many of these

Table 1 — Neural crest tumours

Pheochromocytoma	Oat cell carcinoma
Neuroblastoma	Islet cell tumour
Ganglioneuroma	Merckel cell tumour
Paraganglioma	Schwannoma
Medullary thyroid carcinoma	Neurofibromatosis
Carcinoid	Melanoma

tumours are metabolically active and show the characteristic electron microscopic finding of secretory granules in the cytoplasm. Because of an oxidation process of the intracellular catecholamine stores the chromaffin cells stain dark upon exposure to dichromate salts.

Since 1984 [^{131}I]MIBG has also been used for the diagnosis and treatment of neuroblastoma. This chapter will review the background of this radiopharmaceutical, the basis for its use in therapy of neuroblastoma, and the indications, procedure, preliminary results and side effects published to date.

2. THE COMPOUND

2.1 Development

Most of the work of the development of adrenomedullary radiopharmaceuticals took place at the University of Michigan in Ann Arbor. In 1967 Morales *et al.* [3] first demonstrated that ^{14}C-labelled epinephrine and its precursors concentrated in the adrenal medulla. In 1969 Lieberman *et al.* [4] demonstrated dopamine uptake in the normal human adrenal medulla as well as, in much greater concentrations, in neuroblastoma. Anderson *et al.* [5] subsequently reported [^{14}C]dopamine uptake in phaeochromocytoma. As the ^{14}C label is not suitable for γ-camera imaging, radioiodination of dopamine and its analogues was performed, but the ^{125}I-labelled compounds showed too little uptake in the adrenal medulla to be used for scintigraphic imaging [6].

A second approach, based on the functional similarity between adrenomedullary chromaffin cells and adrenergic neurons, used radiolabelled compounds which have a strong affinity for adrenergic nerves, such as bretylium and guanethidine [7].

Combination of the benzyl group of bretylium with the guanidine group of guanethidine led to a series of aralkylguanidines, which have an even greater antiadrenergic effect [8]. In 1980 Wieland *et al.* [9] compared the ^{125}I-labelled *ortho, para* and *meta* isomers of iodobenzylguanidine in dogs and found the latter two to have a strong affinity for, and a long retention in, the adrenal medulla as well as early high myocardial concentrations . In a subsequent evalution of ^{123}I- and ^{131}I-labelled MIBG in 15 rhesus monkeys [10] this compound, which had initially been regarded to be more suitable as a myocardial imaging agent, showed superior adrenomedullary imaging properties over its *para* isomer. Subcellular fractionation of the dog's adrenal medulla proved that MIBG is mainly sequestered in the storage granules of chromaffin cells.

In the first human studies with [^{131}I]MIBG in 1981 Sisson *et al.* [11] demonstrated successful detection of phaeochromocytoma with this radiopharmaceutical in eight patients, although it became clear that the normal adrenal medulla in man is hardly ever visible on [^{131}I]MIBG scintigrams.

Since then studies with [^{131}I]MIBG around the world have proven the diagnostic efficacy of this compound for the detection of phaeochromocytoma and several other neural crest tumours, and [^{131}I]MIBG is being applied for therapy of some of the malignant tumours in this group.

2.2 Uptake mechanism and metabolism

Although the exact mechanism of uptake of [^{131}I]MIBG remains unclear, it is believed to share the uptake and storage mechanism with norepinephrine, in two ways: a sodium-dependent system with a high affinity but low capacity, which is easily saturable, and a sodium-independent, apparently unsaturable process of passive diffusion [12]. At lower concentrations, as in diagnostic scintigraphy, norepinephrine and MIBG uptake occurs predominantly by the sodium-dependent mechanism, as the uptake can be inhibited by uptake-one inhibitors such as desmethylimipramine and cocaine; at higher concentrations, as in [^{131}I]MIBG therapy, the passive diffusion, which is much less sensitive to the inhibitory effects of these drugs, prevails [13].

Unlike norepinephrine, MIBG is not metabolized by either monoamine oxidase (MAO) or catechol-*O*-methyltransferase (COMT) [14]. HPLC of daily urine samples of eight patients treated with [^{131}I]MIBG for phaeochromocytoma at the University of Michigan [15] showed that the majority of [^{131}I]MIBG is excreted unaltered via the kidneys and that 70–90% of the administered activity was recovered in the urine within 4 days.

2.3 Normal distribution

The normal and abnormal distribution of [^{131}I]MIBG, as visualized by scintigraphy in 84 patients, was described by Nakajo *et al.* [16]. In patients with no clinical, radiological or biochemical evidence of phaeochromocytoma the salivary glands, liver, spleen and urinary bladder were usually visualized, in about half of the cases the heart and lower zones of the lungs were seen, and the colon, upper lung zones and the kidneys appeared less frequently or seldom. The thyroid was only visualized when this organ was indadequately blocked. Normal adrenal glands were seldom visualized by [^{131}I]MIBG scintigraphy: in 2% of the cases they were faintly imaged at 24 h and at 48 h in 16%. However, when [^{131}I]MIBG was used for scintigraphy, the normal adrenal glands were visualized on 24 h images in six out of eight patients [17] because of the greater photon flux and greater sensitivity of gammacameras to ^{123}I emissions.

The myocardial concentration of [^{131}I]MIBG is due to specific uptake in adrenergic neuronal vesicles, as it can be inhibited by reserpine premedication, a blocker of vesicular uptake of norepinephrine. The intensity of [^{131}I]MIBG activity in the heart was found to be inversely correlated with catecholamine levels in serum, suggesting a competition of [^{131}I]MIBG and catecholamines for uptake in myocardial adrenergic neurons [18].

3. THE LABEL

Meta-iodo-benzylguanidine may be labelled with iodine-131, iodine-123 or iodine-125.

Iodine-131 decays by β and γ emission to stable xenon-131 with a physical half-life of 8.04 days. As a label of tumour-seeking radiopharmaceuticals, ^{131}I can be used both for diagnostic scintigraphy and radionuclide therapy of malignant tumours.

Iodine-123, a more recently used cyclotron-produced radionuclide decays always via electron capture to tellurium-123 and emits only γ-rays of which the 159 keV emissions prevail. The physical half-life of 13.3 h, the lack of β particles and the ideal imaging properties make this radionuclide very suitable for diagnostic use (planar scintigraph and single photon emission tomography), but not for delayed imaging and therapy.

Iodine-125 has a physical half-life of 60 days, decays via electron capture (Auger cascade) to tellurium-125 and emits only γ-rays with a 35 keV energy peak and X-rays

(27 keV). Because of the physical properties of this radionuclide, ^{125}I emissions can hardly be visualized with a γ camera in human beings. Therefore iodine-125 is not suitable for diagnostic scintigraphy, but [^{131}I]MIBG is available for investigational use (*in vitro* measurements and autoradiography) and may eventually be used for therapy.

4. DIAGNOSTIC USE OF [^{131}I]MIBG IN NEUROBLASTOMA

At the Netherlands Cancer Institute more than 300 total body scintigrams have been obtained from 78 patients with neuroblastoma by November 1987. 73 of these patients were children with ages of 0–14 years. Scintigrams were made 24, 48 and 72 h after i.v. administration of 18.5–37 MBq (0.5–1 mCi) of [^{131}I]MIBG.

In 13 patients, who were in a complete remission with a normal urinary excretion of catecholamine metabolites, the scintigram was normal. The [^{131}I]MIBG was positive in 62 of 65 patients with documented disease (95.4%). Among these were eight patients with a normal urinalysis for catecholamine metabolites and seven patients with negative bone marrow aspirations, in whom bone marrow invasion was shown scintigraphically. [^{131}I]MIBG scintigraphy correctly demonstrated primary, residual and recurrent tumour masses, as well as diffuse bone marrow infiltration and skeletal, lymph node and soft tissue metastases [19]. In some cases the localization and extent of the disease was shown better by single-photon emission tomography [20].

Cumulative reported findings in the world literature [21], concerning 550 patients with neuroblastoma, indicate that more than 90% of these tumours are able to concentrate [^{131}I]MIBG. Scintigraphy using [^{131}I]MIBG together with urinalysis for catecholamine metabolites are now considered the most sensitive methods for diagnosis, staging and follow up of neuroblastoma.

In our series the tumour concentrations of [^{131}I]MIBG ranged from 0.05% to 10.1% of the net administered dose and the calculated effective half-life at tumour sites varied from 2.6 to 8 days [22]. A good concentration and long retention in the tumour in comparison with normal tissues (Fig. 1) are the basis for therapeutic use of the agent, in analogy with the use of radioiodine in thyroid cancer.

5. THERAPY WITH OPEN SOURCES

The effect of radiation therapy on a tumour depends on the total absorbed radiation dose to which the tumour is exposed and on the sensitivity of the lesion to radiation. The formulation to calculate the absorbed radiation dose delivered by a β-emitting radionuclide which is uniformly distributed and decays within water-equivalent tissue (e.g. the tumour) is

$$D_\beta\,(\mathrm{Gy}) = 19.9 \times C \times E \times T_{1/2}(\mathrm{eff})$$

in which C is the concentration in MBq per gram of tissue, E is the average β energy in MeV and $T_{1/2}$(eff) the effective half-life in days, which accounts for the fixed

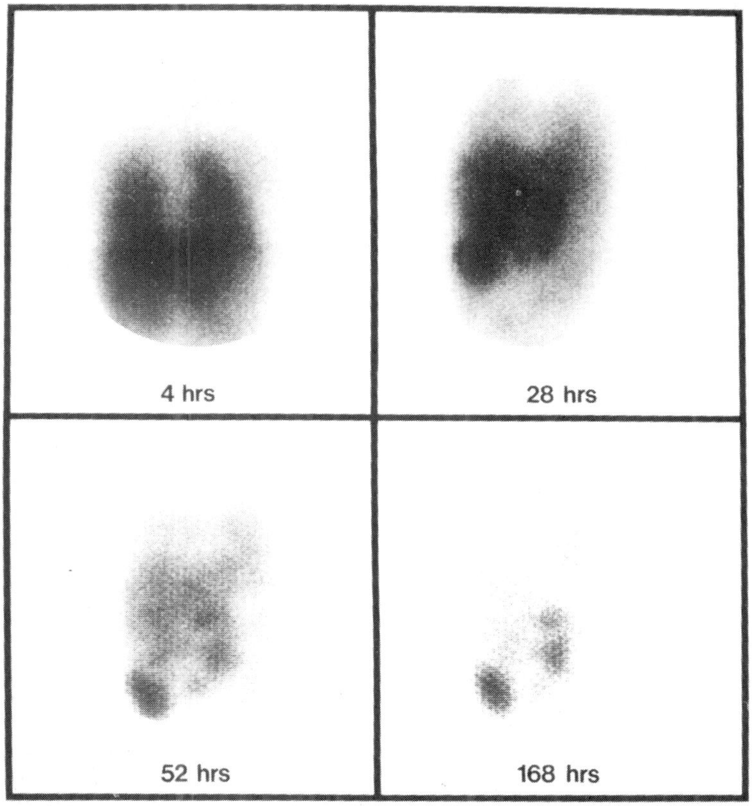

Fig. 1 — Scintigraphic images of a 5-year-old girl with recurrent neuroblastoma below the liver and in the upper abdomen, taken 4, 28, 52 and 168 h after a therapeutic dose of [^{131}I]MIBG and demonstrating the difference in pharmacokinetic behaviour of this compound in the tumour and normal tissues, such as lungs, heart and liver.

physical decay of the radionuclide and an approximation of the biological turnover of the compound, which is variable.

Specificity of localization or a high tumour-to-background ratio is the key factor in delivering radiation to a tumour by means of internally administered radiopharmaceuticals. For tumour targeting various metabolic characteristics and biological properties of tumour cells can be exploited.

Targeting via the metabolic pathway may be the result of an active transport into the tumour cell (e.g. radioiodide transport into thyroid carcinoma), of the use of radiolabelled precursors and metabolites, of metabolic trapping or other means of retention within cells (e.g. the retention of [^{131}I]MIBG in storage vesicles), or of inhibition of the efflux from cells.

To achieve meaningful radiation doses it is essential that the tumour cells have sufficient and accessible binding sites and that the radiopharmaceutical is 'carrier free', i.e. not containing non-labelled molecules which also bind to the target, thereby reducing the number of binding sites available for the radioactive compound.

When the radiolabelled material has reached the target the radiation effect can only be maximally exploited if it remains in that tissue for total decay. In practice this is almost never the case because of biological turnover.

Also, the choice of radionuclide in terms of its physical characteristics plays an important role in the delivery of an adequate radiation dose. Usually low energy β-emitters are preferred, in order to achieve intense irradiation of the target but to spare the surrounding tissues.

As far as handling, tumour response and possible side effects or long-term effects are concerned, [^{131}I]MIBG therapy can best be compared with the use of ^{131}I, which, as iodide, has been applied for treatment of hyperthyroidism, ablation of thyroid remnants after surgery for thyroid carcinoma, and in high doses for irradiation of recurrent or metastatic differentiated carcinoma for over 40 years now. About one million patients worldwide have safely and effectively been treated with ^{131}I doses usually ranging from 110 to 370 MBq (3–10 mCi) for hyperthyroidism [23].

Doses up to 7.4 GBq (200 mCi) are usually applied for ^{131}I treatment of metastatic differentiated thyroid carcinoma. Several series have demonstrated the efficacy of ^{131}I therapy of metastatic thyroid carcinoma in terms of survival [24–26]. Possible acute side effects are nausea and vomiting, sialadenitis, radiation sickness (hardly ever seen at dosages below 7.4 GBq), temporary painful swelling of metastases, and bone marrow suppression. Possible long-term effects of ^{131}I therapy are haematological effects, fertility disorders, induction of leukaemia and other second neoplasms [27].

Major series, in which patients teated with ^{131}I have been followed up for decades, show that side effects and long-term complications of this treatment do not constitute a real problem. Haematological effects appear to be moderate and related to the whole body dose [28]. Sarkar *et al.* [29] found no incidence of decreased fertility or birth abnormalities during follow up (up to 25 years) of 40 children treated with ^{131}I for thyroid cancer. Induction of leukaemia by ^{131}I treatment is extremely rare: 13 of such cases have been reported in the literature [30]. Wiseman *et al.* [31] reported two cases of non-Hodgkin lymphoma developing in the salivary glands 10 and 3 years after ^{131}I therapy for thyroid carcinoma.

6. [^{131}I]MIBG THERAPY

Against this background of more than 40 years experience of ^{131}I therapy for thyroid carcinoma, showing great efficacy and safety of using doses up to 7.4 GBq (200 mCi), the application of [^{131}I]MIBG for the treatment of neural crest tumours, which adequately concentrates this radiopharmaceutical, is a logical step. Although the radiopharmeuctical and the indications are new, as is the fact that in the case of neuroblastoma the majority of patients are children, requiring some adaptations of the logistics of isolation therapy, this form of treatment should not be regarded as experimental, but as a new application of ^{131}I therapy via metabolic targeting, in which MIBG merely acts as a vehicle.

6.1 Indications

For the treatment of neuroblastoma patients with [^{131}I]MIBG two patient groups can be distinguished: (1) those with residual disease, in whom the treatment has a curative intention, and (2) those with progessive, chemotherapy-resistant disease in whom the treatment is given for palliation. Patients are selected upon dosimetric findings in tracer studies, using diagnostic amounts of radioactivity, and the availability of alternative treatment modalities.

6.2 Procedure

For therapeutic purposes [^{131}I]MIBG with a higher specific activity (30–40 mCi/mg instead of 1 mCi/mg) is used. 3.7–7.4 GBq (100–200 mCi) [^{131}I]MIBG, diluted in 100 cm^3 0.9% sodium chloride and mounted in a lead-shielded infusion system, is administered intravenously over 4–24 h at 4–6 week intervals.

Patients are admitted to nuclear-protected hospital isolation facilities for 4–6 days per treatment, dependent on local legislation, and need to use an iodide solution for 2 weeks, starting one day prior to treatment, in order to protect the thyroid from free ^{131}I. Daily scintigrams are made to monitor the pharmacokinetics of the agent *in vivo* and to estimate the absorbed radiation dose to the tumour.

Whenever young children need to be isolated, one of the parents, who during the isolation period can stay in an adjacent room and also has to use the iodide solution, is asked to take care of the child. Continuous monitoring of the external radiation dose to these parents revealed cumulative doses of 0.3–1.25 mSv (30–125 mrem) per treatment dose and the calculated dose equivalent from internal contamination was negligible [32]. This shows that the advantage of having parents participate in the care of their child can be obtained at essentially no increased radiation risk. To overcome the temporary inconvenience of isolation the children are kept busy, e.g. by means of video films.

6.3 Results

Since June 1984 43 patients with neural crest tumours have recieved more than 120 therapeutic doses of [^{131}I]MIBG at The Netherlands Cancer Institute: 30 patients because of neuroblastoma (29 children), 3 for malignant pheochromocytoma, 9 for metastatic carcinoid and 1 with medullary thyroid carcinoma.

After children had received 1.85 GBq (50 mCi) initially and subsequently 3.7 GBq (100 mCi), at present 7.4 GBq (200 mCi) is administered as a first dose, followed by 3.7 GBq (100 mCi) doses thereafter. With this regimen the following results were obtained in neuroblastoma patients:

(1) 5 complete remissions: 4 of these patients, however, had a relapse 5–23 months after the start of [^{131}I]MIBG therapy and 2 could then again be treated with [^{131}I]MIBG; the fifth patient died 3 months after the end of [^{131}I]MIBG treatment as a result of a cerebral haemorrhage during persistent thrombocytopaenia; as at autopsy no tumour was found, we regard this as a toxic death.
(2) 13 partial remissions: i.e. a greater than 50% decrease in tumour volume in 7 patients and considerable scintigraphic improvement in 6 other patients with non-measurable lesions.
(3) 6 patients with stable disease (i.e. no change).
(4) 5 patients with progression of disease. One patient was lost to follow up.

It should be noted that most of these patients had progressive stage IV neuroblastoma and were only treated with [^{131}I]MIBG after all other treatment modalities had been used.

At a symposium on the use of [^{131}I]MIBG in neuroblastoma in Rome, September 1986, data from 80 neuroblastoma patients treated with [^{131}I]MIBG around the world were gathered and published: adding up the experience of the major groups at that point [33–39], concerning 64 evaluable patients including the initial 18 from Amsterdam, discussed above, the following figures for documented response are obtained: 4 complete remissions, 27 partial remissions, no change or stabilization of disease in 21 and progressive disease in 12 patients. These figures are encouraging, if one considers that most of these patients had stage IV, progressive and intensively pretreated disease.

Figs. 2 and 3 show examples of a complete response and a good partial remission respectively in two neuroblastoma patients treated with [^{131}I]MIBG.

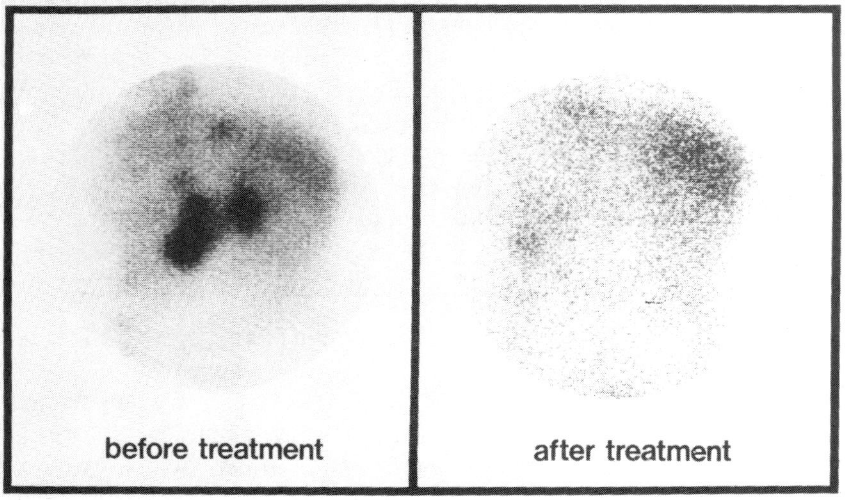

Fig. 2 — Scintigrams at 67 h after administration of [^{131}I]MIBG in a 22-year-old boy with recurrent paraspinal neuroblastoma before and after successful [^{131}I]MIBG therapy leading to complete remission.

6.4 Side effects

In an evaluation of side effects in 23 patients, who were treated with [^{131}I]MIBG for neuroblastoma in our institute [40], haematological effects of [^{131}I]MIBG treatment were observed in 19 patients, with a predominance of the occurrence of thrombocytopaenia. As is shown in Fig. 4, in some patients the onset of thrombocytopaenia was immediately after the first dose, whereas other patients only develop a decrease in platelet counts after successive therapy doses (cumulative toxicity).

The bone marrow status was found to have an important influence on the haematological side effects: in 2 of 3 patients who never had demonstrated any sign

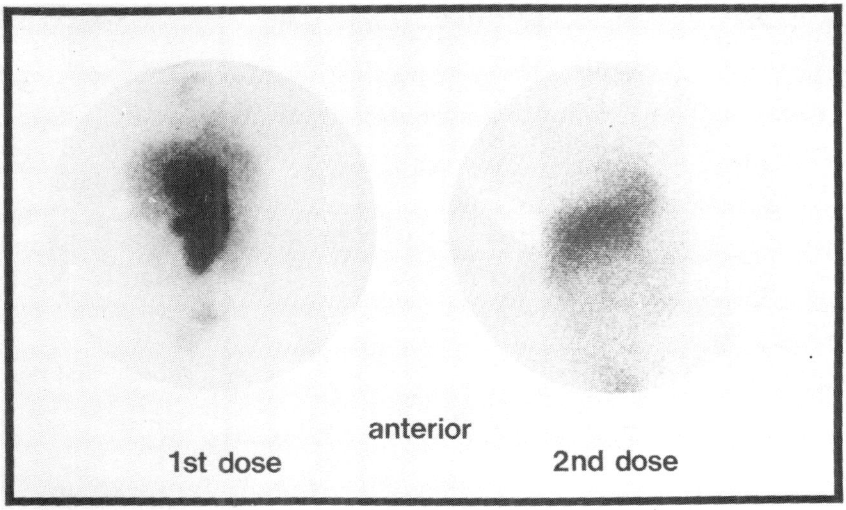

Fig. 3 — Good partial remission (i.e >90% decrease in tumour volume) after a single dose of 7.4 GBq (200 mCi) of [^{131}I]MIBG in a 4-year-old girl with progressive metastatic neuroblastoma.

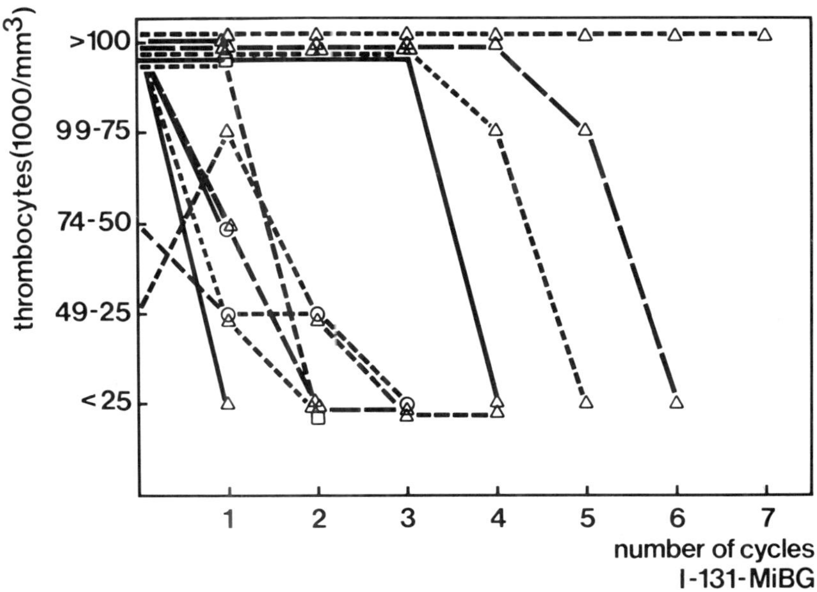

Fig. 4 — Thrombocyte counts of neuroblastoma patients undergoing [^{131}I]MIBG therapy.

of bone marrow involvement no side effects occurred; 6 patients who, at the time of [^{131}I]MIBG treatment, showed no bone marrow disease, but previously had been proven to have invaded bone marrow, had thrombocytopaenia only; however, 11 of 12 patients, who, during [^{131}I]MIBG therapy, revealed bone marrow involvement, developed severe bone marrow depressions. As is shown by Fig. 5, in patients with

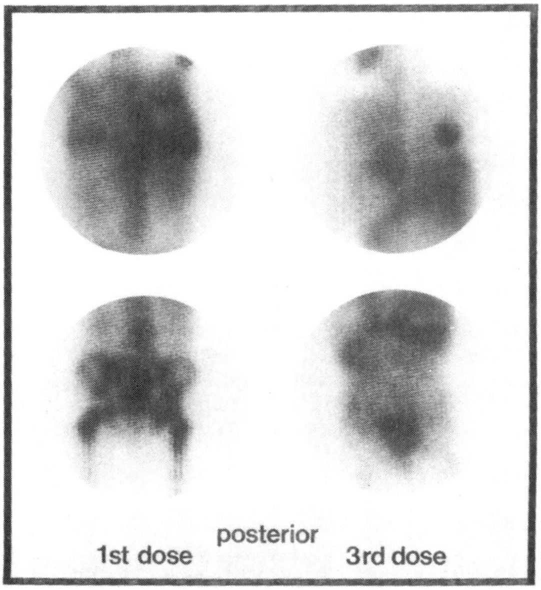

Fig. 5 — Post-therapeutic scintigrams of a 5-year-old boy treated with [^{131}I]MIBG for a large rib lesion and presenting clinically unsuspected bone marrow involvement (left): after three successive doses the tumour is gone and the bone marrow is cleared; however, severe bone marrow depression occurred (the thoracic accumulation of activity on both scintigrams is due to a residue of the dose in the porth a cath system).

bone marrow involvement the bone marrow may be cleared by [^{131}I]MIBG therapy, but this practically always results in severe bone marrow toxicity, and should only be anticipated when salvage methods are available.

In two patients impairment of renal function (increase of serum creatinine and decrease of creatinine clearance) was found after treatment with [^{131}I]MIBG. In most cases, however, no detrimental effect to the kidneys was found. As most of these patients had been treated with high doses of Cisplatin and some of them already had disturbances of renal function at the start of [^{131}I]MIBG treatment, it was difficult to assess whether any nephrotoxic effect can be attributed to [^{131}I]MIBG. However, in one patient, who had only one remaining kidney, we have observed that impairment of renal function, which had been induced by preceding chemotherapy with Cisplatin, was enhanced after [^{131}I]MIBG therapy, as is shown in Fig. 6.

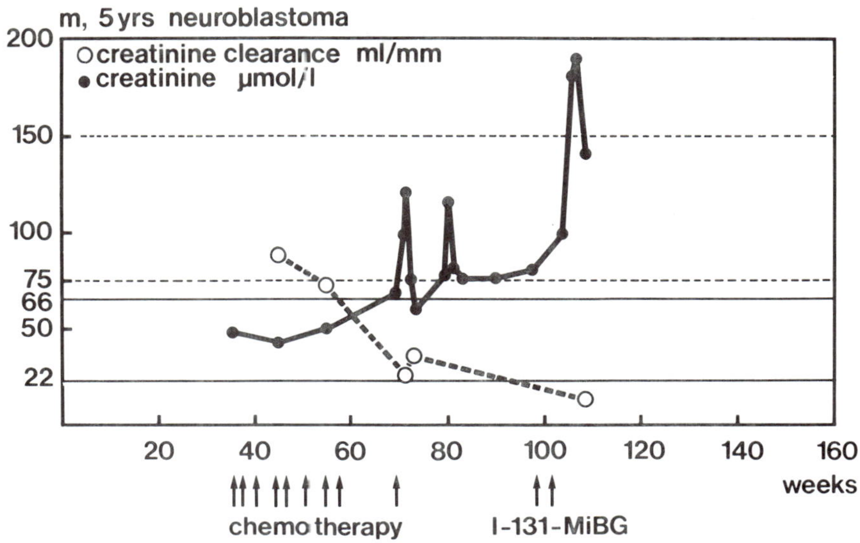

Fig. 6 — Serum creatinine levels and creatinine clearance in a 5-year-old boy with neuroblastoma, during treatment with Cisplatin and [^{131}I]MIBG, showing further deterioration of renal function after [^{131}I]MIBG superimposed on Cisplatin-induced nephropathy.

Apart from occasional nausea on the day after the [^{131}I]MIBG infusion no gastrointestinal, hepatic and cardiac side effects have been recorded.

7. CONCLUSION

[^{131}I]MIBG treatment is an effective treatment in neuroblastoma and can be used safely in patients with residual disease without bone marrow involvement at any stage of their disease. Major toxicity can be expected when the bone marrow is invaded due to irreparable radiation damage to bone marrow stem cells, especially to the megakaryocytes. In these patients [^{131}I]MIBG can be used as a palliative treatment to relieve pain, but haematological toxicity must be accepted.

REFERENCES

[1] Shapiro, B., Copp, J. E., Sisson, J. C., Eyre, P. L., Wallis, J. & Beierwaltes, W. H. (1985). Iodine-131 metaiodobenzylguanidine for the locating of suspected pheochromocytoma: experience in 400 cases. *J. Nucl. Med.* **26** 576–585

[2] Sisson, J. C., Shapiro, B., Beierwaltes, W. H., Glowniak, J. V., Nakajo, M., Mangner, T. J., Carey, J. E., Swanson, D. P., Copp, J. E., Satterlee, W. G. & Wieland, D. M. (1984). Radiopharmaceutical treatment of malignant pheochromocytoma. *J. Nucl. Med.* **25** 197–206

[3] Morales, J. O., Beierwaltes, W. H., Counsell, R. E. & Meier, D. E. (1967). The concentration of radioactivity from labeled epinephrine and its precursors in the dog adrenal medulla. *J. Nucl. Med.* **8** 800–809

[4] Lieberman, L. M., Beierwaltes, W. H., Varma, V. M., Weinhold, P. & Ling, R. (1969). Labeled dopamine concentration in human adrenal medulla and in neuroblastoma. *J. Nucl. Med.* **10** 93–97
[5] Anderson, B. G., Beierwaltes, W. H., Harrison, T. S., Ansari, A. N., Buswink, A. A. & Ice, R. D. (1973). Labeled dopamine concentration in pheochromocytomas. *J. Nucl. Med.* **14** 781–784
[6] Ice, R. D., Wieland, D. M., Beierwaltes, W. H., Lawton, R. G. & Redmond, M. J. (1975). Concentration of dopamine analogs in the adrenal medulla. *J. Nucl. Med.* **16** 1147–1151
[7] Korn, N., Buswink, A., Yu, T., Carr, E. A., Caroll, M. & Counsell, R. E. (1977). A radioiodinated bretylium analog as a potential agent for scanning the adrenal medulla. *J. Nucl. Med.* **18** 87–89
[8] Short, J. H. & Darby, T. D. (1967). Sympathetic nervous system blocking agents. III. Derivatives of benzylguanidine. *J. Med. Chem.* **10** 833–840
[9] Wieland, D. M., Wu, J. L., Brown, L. E., Mangner, T. J., Swanson, D. P. & Beierwaltes, W. M. (1980). Radiolabeled adrenergic neuron blocking agents: adrenomedullary imaging with [^{131}I]iodobenzylguanidine. *J. Nucl. Med.* **21** 349–353
[10] Wieland, D. M., Brown, L. E., Tobes, M. C., Rogers, W. L., Marsh, D. D., Mangner, T. J., Swanson, D. P. & Beierwaltes, W. H. (1981). Imaging the primate adrenal medulla with [^{123}I] and [^{131}I]metaiodobenzylguanidine: concise communication. *J. Nucl. Med.* **22** 358–364
[11] Sisson, J. C., Frager, M. S., Valk, T. W., Gross, M. D., Swanson, D. P., Wieland, D. M., Tobes, M. C., Beierwaltes, W. H. & Thompson, N. W. (1981). Scintigraphic localization of pheochromocytoma. *N. Engl. J. Med.* **305** 12–17
[12] Jaques, S. Jr., Tobes, M. C., Sisson, J. C. & Baker, J. A. (1984). Mechanisms of uptake of norepinephrine (NE) and meta-iodobenzylguanidine (MIBG) into cultured human pheochromocytoma cells. *J. Nucl. Med.* **25** 122
[13] Tobes, M. C., Jaques, S. Jr., Sisson, J. C. & Wieland, D. M. (1984). Mechanisms of uptake of norepinephrine (NE) and meta-iodobenzylguanidine (MIBG) into cultured bovine adrenomedullary cells. *J. Nucl. Med.* **25** 124
[14] Wieland, D. M., Brown, L. E., Rogers, W. L., Worthington, K. C., Wu, J. L., Clinthorn, N. H., Otto, C. A., Swanson, D. P. & Beierwaltes, W. H. (1981). Myocardial imaging with a radioiodinated norepinephrine storage analog. *J. Nucl. Med.* **22** 22–31
[15] Mangner, T. J., Tobes, M. C., Wieland, D. W., Sisson, J. C. & Shapiro, B. (1986). Metabolism of iodine-131 metaiodobenzylguanidine in patients with metastatic pheochromocytoma. *J. Nucl. Med.* **27** 37–44
[16] Nakajo, M., Shapiro, B., Copp, J., Kalff, V., Gross, M. D., Sisson, J. C. & Beierwaltes, W. H. (1983). The normal and abnormal distribution of the adrenomedullary imaging agent *m*-[^{131}I]iodobenzylguanidine I-131 MIBG in man: evaluation by scintigraph. *J. Nucl. Med.* **24** 672–682
[17] Lynn, M. D., Shapiro, B., Sisson, J. C., Swanson, D. P., Mangner, T. J., Wieland, D. M., Meyers, L. J., Glowniak, J. V. & Beierwaltes, W. H. (1984). Portrayal of pheochromocytoma and normal human adrenal medulla by *m*[^{123}I]iodobenzylguanidine: concise communication. *J. Nucl. Med.* **25** 436–440

[18] Nakajo, M., Shapiro, B., Glowniak, J., Sisson, J. C. & Beierwaltes, W. H. (1983). Inverse relationship between cardiac accumulation of meta-[^{131}I]-iodobenzylguanidine I-131 MIBG and circulating catecholamines in suspected pheochromocytoma. *J. Nucl. Med.* **24** 1127–1134
[19] Hoefnagel, C. A., Voûte, P. A., de Kraker, J. & Marcuse, H. R. (1987). Radionuclide diagnosis and treatment of neural crest tumours using iodine-131-meta-iodobenzylguanidine. *J. Nucl. Med.* **28** 308–314
[20] Hoefnagel, C. A., Klumper, A. & Voûte, P. A. (1987). Single photon emission tomography using meta-[^{131}I]-iodobenzylguanidine in malignant pheochromocytoma and neuroblastoma: case reports. *J. Med. Imag.* **1** 57–60
[21] Gelfand, M. J. & Hoefnagel, C. A. (1988). In: *Textbook of Pediatric Radiology,* in press
[22] Hoefnagel, C. A., Voûte, P. A., de Kraker, J. & Marcuse, H. R. (1985). Total body scintigraphy with I-131-meta-iodobenzylguanidine for detection of neuroblastoma. *Diagn. Imag. Clin. Med.* **54** 21–27
[23] Becker, D. V. (1982) Radioactive iodine (^{131}I) in the treatment of hyperthyroidism. In: C. H. Beckers (ed.) *Thyroid Diseases,* Pergamon, pp. 145–158
[24] Beierwaltes, W. H., Nishiyama, R. H., Thompson, N. W., Copp, J. E. & Kubo, A. (1982). Survival time and "cure" in papillary and follicular thyroid carcinoma with distant metastases: statistics following University of Michigan therapy. *J. Nucl. Med.* **23** 561–568
[25] Hundeshagen, H. (1983). Postoperative diagnosis and therapy of thyroid carcinoma by nuclear medicine. *Eur. J. Nucl. Med.* **8** 541–545
[26] Creutzig, H., Funke-Voelkers, R., Kroenke, C., Guth, B., Henning, A. & Mueller, S. T. (1987). Risk factors in differentiated thyroid cancer. *J. Nucl. Med.* **28** 576
[27] Freitas, J. E., Gross, M. D., Ripley, S. & Shapiro, B. (1985) Radionuclide diagnosis and therapy of thyroid cancer: current status report. *Semin. Nucl. Med.* **15** 106–131
[28] Sisson, J. C., Hutchinson, R., Johnston, J. Mallette, S., Carey, J., Shapiro, B. & Beierwaltes, W. H. (1987). Acute toxicity of therapeutic I-131-MIBG relates more to whole body than to blood radiation dosimetry. *J. Nucl. Med.* **28** 618
[29] Sarkar, S. D., Beierwaltes, W. H., Gill, S. P. & Cowley, B. J. (1976). Subsequent fertility and birth histories of children and adolescents treated with 131-I for thyroid cancer. *J. Nucl. Med.* **17** 460–464
[30] Hurley, R. J. & Becker, D. V. (1983). The use of radioiodine in the management of thyroid cancer. In: L. M. Freeman & H. S. Weissman (eds.) *Nuclear Medicine Annual 1983,* Raven Press, New York, pp. 348–349
[31] Wiseman, J. C., Halls, I. B. & Joasoo, A. (1982). Two cases of lymphoma of the parotid gland following ablative radioiodine therapy for thyroid carcinoma. *Clin. Endocrinol.* **17** 85–89
[32] Van der Steen, J., Maessen, H. J. M., Hoefnagel, C. A. & Marcuse, H. R. (1986). Radiation protection during therapy with unsealed sources at young children. *Health Phys.* **50** 512–522
[33] Beierwaltes, W. H. (1987). Update on basic research and clinical experience with metaiodobenzylguanidine. *Med. Ped. Oncol.* **15** 163–169
[34] Voûte, P. A., Hoefnagel, C. A., de Kraker, J., Evans, A. E., Hayes, A. &

Green, A. (1987). Radionuclide therapy of neural crest tumors. *Med. Ped. Oncol.* **15** 192–195

[35] Fischer, M., Wehinger, H., Kraus, C., Ritter, J. & Schroeter, W. (1987). Treatment of neuroblastoma with metaiodobenzylguanidine: experience of the Muenster/Kassel group. *Med. Ped. Oncol.* **15** 196–198

[36] Treuner, J., Klingebiel, T. H., Bruchelt, G., Feine, U. & Neithammer, D. (1987). Treatment of neuroblastoma with ^{131}I-metaiodobenzylguanidine: results and side effects. *Med. Ped. Oncol.* **15** 199–202

[37] Bestagno, M., Guerra, P., Puricelli, G. P., Colombo, L. & Calculli, G. (1987) Treatment of neuroblastoma with ^{131}I-metaiodobenzylguanidine: the experience of an Italian study group. *Med. Ped. Oncol.* **15** 203–204

[38] Hartmann, O., Lumbroso, J., Lemerle, J., Schlumberger, M., Ricard, M., Aubert, B., Coornaert, S., Merlin, L., Olive, D., De Lumley, L. & Parmentier, C. (1987). Therapeutic use of ^{131}I-metaiodobenzylguanidine (MIBG) in neuroblastoma: a phase II study in nine patients. *Med. Ped. Oncol.* **15** 205–211

[39] Troncone, L., Riccardi, R., Montemaggi, P., Rufini, V., Lasorella, A. & Mastrangelo, R. (1987). Treatment of neuroblastoma with ^{131}I-metaiodobenzylguanidine. *Med. Ped. Oncol.* **15** 220–223

[40] Voûte, P. A., Hoefnagel, C. A., de Kraker, J. & Majoor, M. (1987). Side effects of treatment with I-131-meta-iodobenzylguanidine (I-131-MIBG) in neuroblastoma patients. In: A. E. Evans (ed.) *Advances in Neuroblastoma Research,* Vol. 4, Alan R. Liss, New York, in press

9

Surgery for neuroblastoma

Edward M. Kiely
Department of Paediatric Surgery, Hospital for Sick Children, Great Ormond Street, London WC1N 3JH, UK

1. INTRODUCTION

The role of surgery in the mangement of neuroblastoma has changed. Previously only those with localized disease were amenable to surgery. Now even children who present with advanced and metastatic disease may come within the remit of the surgeon. Metastases may be obliterated by chemotherapy leaving a shrunken, fibrotic, primary tumour to be excised. These operations are usually very difficult and demand considerable commitment and patience on the part of the surgeon who attempts excision. Complete or near-complete excision is now possible for the majority of patients who present with neuroblastoma.

2. ROLE OF SURGERY

The role of surgery may be classed as diagnostic and therapeutic. The latter role may be subdivided into palliative and excisional surgery. The surgeon's role in the provision of long-term vascular access is not within the scope of this chapter.

2.1 Diagnostic surgery

This includes tumour biopsy for diagnosis and staging. Tissue is sometimes required for diagnosis when urine catecholamine excretion is normal and when bone marrow aspirates and trephines are unhelpful. Closed or open biopsies are suitable, but the latter provide larger specimens and are often preferred by pathologists.

Closed biopsies are performed under general anaesthesia using biopsy needles which provide a core of tissue. Because neuroblastomas are often soft and necrotic the tissue sample obtained may be disappointingly small. A delay of several days may then ensue as efforts are made to reach a diagnosis before recourse is made to an open procedure. Parents sometimes find this sequence of events intolerable.

Open biopsies should be performed with an eye to future surgery. An incision is used which can later be extended at the time of the definitive procedure. Because the biopsy sample is larger, diagnostic difficulties are minimized.

In general, open biopsy is preferred for the reasons stated above. However, for some patients the type of disease may indicate which method is preferred. Patients with Evans' stage IVS disease may have accessible skin nodules or, alternatively, massive hepatomegaly. Under these circumstances the type of biopsy indicated is obvious. Finally, in expert hands, endoscopic biopsy in the chest or abdomen may provide enough material for diagnosis.

Local facilities, the availability of electron microscopy and histochemistry may dictate the amount of material needed for diagnosis. The desire to avoid a diagnostic thoracotomy or laparotomy may not be in the patient's interest.

2.2 Palliative surgery

With neuroblastoma, palliative surgery is not simply carried out to relieve symptoms in the absence of cure. It is often performed to alleviate symptoms or to preserve function with every prospect of a final cure. Two forms of palliative surgery are well known — laminectomy to relieve spinal cord compression and abdominal patching in stage IVS disease. In both cases, the need for surgery is not as clearly defined as before. Chemotherapy may be as effective in the majority of cases, thereby avoiding a sizeable procedure. Only where chemotherapy fails is surgery likely to be required.

Massive hepatomegaly in stage IVS disease responds slowly to chemotherapy and a period of positive pressure ventilation may be necessary. Radiotherapy is often used in conjunction with chemotherapy under these circumstances and only when liver growth is unremitting is an abdominal wall patch required. Dacron-backed silastic sheeting is most frequently used but usually detaches after 7–10 days, leaving an open, granulating wound. This may subsequently require formal closure when the liver has regressed in size.

2.3 Excisional surgery

The aim is to remove all visible tumour. This is usually possible in localized disease (Evan's stages I and II), but not always in advanced disease (Evan's stages III and IV). Pre-operative imaging by ultrasound, computerized tomography and magnetic resonance imaging is helpful in estimating the magnitude of the proposed procedure. No reliance should be placed on imaging techniques in assessing resectability.

The attitude of the surgeon will determine the success of the operation. These operations are usually difficult. In addition, the entire procedure may be difficult. The tumour often invades the tunica adventitia of major vessels but rarely involves the tunica media. Consequently it is usually possible to excise extensive tumours and leave the great vessels and their branches intact. There is no alternative to knife dissection. Attempts at blunt or scissors dissection will result in vascular injury. What is required, therefore, is patient, sharp dissection between the adventitia and media of a series of major blood vessels over a period of several hours. Under these circumstances it is easy to consider an individual tumour inoperable. Finally, optical magnification is a considerable asset in precise dissection.

2.4 Abdominal neuroblastoma

The principle of the operation is to isolate and preserve the major blood vessels and viscera, and then to remove the tumour. The procedure described here is for extensive abdominal neuroblastoma. The operation is scaled down as necessary for smaller lesions. The surgery is performed under intubated general anaesthesia with muscle relaxation. Continuous arterial and venous pressure monitoring through indwelling cannulae is helpful. In addition a large bore venous cannula above the diaphragm is necessary for volume replacement. A bladder catheter is inserted and the child is placed on a heating blanket. The limbs may also be wrapped to reduce heat loss further. A roll under the lumbar spine may be used to elevate the costal margin with upper abdominal tumours. Prophylactic antibiotics are not used.

The abdomen is opened through a long, transverse upper abdominal incision. A full laparotomy is performed and tumour extent is assessed. The majority of tumours arise in one or other adrenal gland and the dissection commences on this side. The colon is reflected medially together with its blood supply and mesocolon. Care is necessary during reflection of the peritoneum to avoid opening the perinephric fascia. If the peritoneum is invaded by tumour then that portion is left attached. This phase of the dissection is complete when the midline is reached. On the left side it may be necessary to reflect the spleen and pancreas as well. The intestine and all mobilized viscera are placed in a plastic bag, which prevents drying and trauma to the serosal surfaces.

The tumour dissection than commences just distal to the lower margin of the tumour. The external iliac vein on the right side or the external iliac artery on the left side is exposed. The dissection starts more proximally with less extensive tumours. The assistant and operator each pick up adventitia which is incised longitudinally to enter the plane beneath the adventitia. The vessel is dissected circumferentially and the plane of future dissection is estimated. The operator now proceeds proximally in similar fashion — cutting down along the line of the blood vessel until the correct level is reached. The entire circumference of the blood vessel is then exposed and the dissection again proceeds proximally. Usually 1–2cm lengths of vessel are dealt with each time. Once the inferior vena cava (IVC) or aorta are reached the lumbar vessels are encountered and these are usually easily preserved.

On the left side the first visceral branch encountered is the inferior mesenteric artery. This artery may be exposed proximally or distally in the sigmoid mesocolon. The technique remains the same and the proximal few centimetres of vessel may need to be cleared of tumour. The great vessel exposure continues as before until the level of the renal vessels is reached.

The left renal vein is commonly embedded in tumour. There are no special techniques to help expose this vessel. It may be possible to display the junction of the left renal vein with the IVC but frequently this area is also surrounded by tumour. The usual method is to incise the tumour as before along the line of the aorta. The bluish tinge of the left renal vein is usually noted before the wall is breached. In fact, injury to the vein is distinctly unusual. The vein is then dissected over most of its length until it can be freely retracted. If the vein must be sacrificed, the kidney will survive provided that it is not mobilized from its bed. The aortic dissection may then proceed.

The renal arteries are encountered at this level also and just proximally is the origin of the superior mesenteric artery (SMA). The pace of the operation slows considerably at this stage, as every effort is made to avoid vascular injury. It may be easier to expose the left side of the aorta above the left renal artery and then to dissect transversely towards the SMA. Once the root of the vessel has been displayed the rest of its dissection is completed as before.

On the right side the IVC and renal veins are displayed. Care is necessary in mobilizing the posterior aspect of the IVC as the right renal artery is very close. There are no branches of note above this level until the right adrenal vein is encountered. This is often a sizeable structure. The IVC is dissected free circumferentially until a curved vascular clamp can be applied to the side of the IVC. Care is necessary above the level of the adrenal vein as hepatic veins may enter close by. Normally, however, the clamp can be applied and the vein transected without difficulty. The defect in the IVC is closed with a running 5/0 vascular suture.

On the left side the aortic dissection proceeds above the SMA. The left adrenal artery is cauterized or ligated. If the tumour is central there may be a substantial blood supply directly from the aorta at this level. The coeliac axis is encountered just above the SMA at the level of the median arcuate ligament. It is exposed as before if possible. Sometimes tumour bulk dictates a different approach. Retrograde dissection along the splenic artery may be easier. When the main trunk has been exposed the splenic, left gastric and hepatic arteries are displayed in turn. The two branches to the diaphragm are sacrificed.

The major part of the dissection is now complete, although no tumour has been removed. The primary tumour is usually excised at this point. It may have a substantial blood supply from the diaphragm and posterior abdominal wall and many bleeding points will need electrocautery. The tumour may need to be dissected free from the kidney but renal invasion is unusual.

Once the primary tumour has been removed nodal disease remains. Renal hilar invasion is common and painstaking dissection is required to remove all tumour and to preserve the kidney. The renal artery and its branches are freed in turn and then the renal vein and its branches. Nephrectomy will occasionally be necessary to achieve tumour clearance. Present-day chemotherapy is nephrotoxic and nephrectomy may reduce renal function to a dangerous degree. It is well worthwhile persisting with dissection in the renal hilum to avoid the need for later dialysis or renal transplantation.

Removal of nodes lateral to the great vessels is usually fairly straightforward. The lumbar vessels may be damaged at some distance from their origins, but as many as possible are preserved. The ureters are rarely involved by tumour and are not usually at risk. Removal of tumour from between and behind the great vessels is more difficult but not unduly hazardous. Invasion of the vertebral bodies has not been encountered and the tumour is readily freed from the spine.

Tumour in the lesser sac presents particular problems. Both aorta and IVC must be dissected which means reflection of colon on either side, together with the spleen and pancreas. When the major visceral branches have been displayed the portal triad is dissected free. The duodenum and head of pancreas are lifted anteriorly to free the posterior aspect of the pancreas and the superior mesenteric vein. The tumour is then ready for removal with attached right crus of diaphragm.

Considerable haemorrhage may occur throughout the procedure. This is mainly from cut tumour surfaces. Once the tumour has been removed, there is remarkably little bleeding. There is often heavy lymphatic leakage, however, which is not amenable to suturing or electrocautery. Symptomatic chylous ascites has not, so far, been encountered after one of these operations. Once haemostasis has been secured, any defects in the mesocolon are repaired and the gut is replaced within the abdomen. The colon is not sutured in place and no drains are used.

2.5 Mediastinal tumours

The same principle applies — identify and preserve vital structures and then remove the tumour. In addition to the blood vessels, however, the oesophagus, trachea, recurrent laryngeal and phrenic nerves must be preserved. In practice these structures rarely intrude. Even the major blood vessels are usually at a safe distance from the tumour. However, the tumour may extend posteriorly through one or more intercostal spaces and partial rib resection may be necessary to maximize tumour clearance.

2.6 Neuroblastomas at other sites

Laminectomy is outside the scope of this surgeon and this chapter. Excision of cervical and pelvic tumours follows the basic principles outlined above.

2.7 Post-operative care

Vascular monitoring is continued for a minimum of 24 h. Volume replacement to compensate for lymphatic and other losses into the abdomen may be considerable. We use plasma as necessary. Blood glucose monitoring is also performed 4–6 hourly. Continuous narcotic infusion is used to provide analgesia. Otherwise post-operative care is similar to that for any other major laparotomy.

3. RESULTS

The author's experience with neuroblastoma is limited to 60 cases over the past four years. 53 of these were patients with stage IV disease undergoing surgery after several courses of chemotherapy. With increasing experience there has been a trend towards more complete excision. Only two cases of vascular invasion have been encountered — one venous and one arterial. In all other cases, tumour growth did not involve the tunica media. These patients had unresectable tumours. Two had obvious fresh tumour growth and excision was not attempted. The third has a heavily calcified tumour which could not be incised.

One operative death has occurred from hypoglycaemia. This 4-year-old boy had a 10 h procedure and a 5 l blood transfusion for removal of a large, upper abdominal neuroblastoma. At that time blood glucose levels were not routinely measured and he developed severe hypoglycaemia 24 h after surgery. He sustained catastrophic brain damage and died five days later. No tumour was found in his abdomen at autopsy. The fall in blood sugar was probably related to the massive transfusion. The dextrose load with the infused blood resulted in a rebound hypoglycaemia. We have encountered a lesser fall (to 2.5 mmol/l) in a second child since then. This was rapidly corrected by 10% dextrose infusion.

A consistent finding in those who have had extensive arterial dissections has been the development of post-operative diarrhoea. On occasion this has been severe enough to delay further treatment. When the coeliac axis, SMA and inferior mesenteric artery have been 'cleaned', the gut is denervated. The long-term results of this are unknown but, at least in the short term, diarrhoea is a problem. Spontaneous improvement in bowel habit occurs but several children have frequent, loose stools more than two years after surgery. Loperamide has been of considerable help to these children.

Of greater concern is the possibility that boys may be rendered impotent by extensive distal aortic dissection. The presacral nerve is preserved where possible but, frequently, the distal aorta and common iliac arteries are clean at the end of the procedure. The consequences for girls are also not clear. One should, therefore, try to steer a course between adequate clearance and preservation of a vital structure.

At present, the incidence of post-operative adhesion obstruction is about 5%. The rates might well be higher if all patients survived.

The most recent survival figures for advanced (stages III and IV) neuroblastoma from this hospital cover the years 1979 to 1985. 90 patients presented in that time, 11 with stage III and 70 with stage IV disease. 83 patients survived long enough for surgery to be considered — usually after four to eight courses of chemotherapy. Of 37 who had more than 75% of the primary tumour excised, 14 survived more than one year disease free. Of 29 who had less than a 75% resection or who did not undergo surgery, only one survived 12 months disease free.

4. CONCLUSION

The role of surgery in neuroblastoma is diagnostic and therapeutic. It appears that a greater proportion of patients with advanced disease is now curable. This is mainly due to improving chemotherapy. The therapeutic effectiveness of surgery is unclear owing to constantly changing drug regimens. Surgery of course is curative in localized disease. From the figures quoted above, surgery does appear to influence survival on advanced disease also. At present, it is not known whether 95% excision of residual tumour is better than 75% excision. Perhaps the characteristics of individual tumours allow for more complete resection is some than in others. However, chemotherapy has presented surgeons with a new challenge — contracted fibrous tumours enveloping a series of essential structures. The majority of these tumours are amenable to resection. For the foreseeable future, that is the role of surgery in neuroblastoma.

ACKNOWLEDGEMENT

I am grateful to Dr. Jon Pritchard, whose patients these are, for providing the results quoted above.

Index